A Study of the Lack of
HIV/AIDS Awareness
among African American
Women: A Leadership
Perspective

AWARENESS THAT ALL CULTURES SHOULD KNOW ABOUT

by
Betty L. Ragsdale-Hearns

A Dissertation Presented in Partial Fulfillment of the Requirements
for the Degree DOCTOR OF MANAGEMENT
IN ORGANIZATIONAL LEADERSHIP

UNIVERSITY OF PHOENIX
October 2011

Order this book online at www.trafford.com
or email orders@trafford.com

Most Trafford titles are also available at major online book retailers.

Printed in the United States of America.

ISBN: 978-1-4669-4852-5 (sc)
ISBN: 978-1-4669-4851-8 (hc)
ISBN: 978-1-4669-4853-2 (e)

Library of Congress Control Number: 2012913065

Trafford rev. 07/26/2012

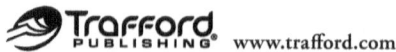 www.trafford.com

North America & international
toll-free: 1 888 232 4444 (USA & Canada)
phone: 250 383 6864 ♦ fax: 812 355 4082

A STUDY OF THE LACK OF HIV/AIDS AWARENESS AMONG AFRICAN AMERICAN WOMEN: A LEADERSHIP PERSPECTIVE

By

Betty L. Ragsdale

October 2011

Approved:

Alex Kadrie, Ph.D., Mentor
Mary Jo Brinkman, Ph.D., Committee Member
Ronald Black, Ed.D., Committee Member

Accepted and Signed: _____ _____
                          Alex Kadrie, Ph.D.   Date

Accepted and Signed: _____ _____
                          Mary Jo Brinkman, Ph.D.   Date

Accepted and Signed: _____ _____
                          Ronald Black, Ed.D.   Date

_____ _____
Jeremy Moreland, Ph.D.   Date
Dean, School of Advanced Studies
University of Phoenix

ABSTRACT

This qualitative grounded theory study focused on a leadership perspective about HIV/AIDS awareness involving 30 African American women who were participants in this research study from Dallas and Fort Worth areas of Texas. The problem is that African American women are not aware of the social contact of the HIV/AIDS disease, which is important to understanding the leader's perspectives of the affects the disease has on their community. The purpose of the current study was to explore the lack of HIV/AIDS awareness in African American women. Interviews were conducted through semi-structured questionnaires; grounded theory methodology was used to generate a theory of how the participants gave meaning to HIV/AIDS awareness. Results revealed participants are not aware of leader's commitment to educate the community. The theoretical model included personal context, support and education, socio-cultural meaning, and personal meaning, all of which related to the formation of a global meaning regarding HIV/AIDS awareness. The significant themes, which emerged from participant data, indicated the leaders influence on the African American community and participant's awareness about HIV/AIDS. The issues were discussed as the emergent theoretical model and its components, which included implications of research, practice, stigma, burden, advocacy, and awareness. Leadership, education, and community resources were the dominant themes that emerged in the study. The study findings imply an increased need for leaders to present public awareness about the affects HIV/AIDS has on the African American community. Future research should consider the explicit nature of the answers, which benefited the study. The information would be helpful while improving the quality of life available for African American women, and would enable leaders to interact with a leadership perspective (USAID, 2009).

DEDICATION

This work is dedicated to God for strength and assurance; then to my children, Crystal and Monica Ragsdale; to my grandchildren: Crysten Kelly, Olivia Hadnot, and Darren Landon Kelly; and to the Glory of God. One generation shall praise thy works to another, and shall declare thy mighty acts (Psalm 145:4, KJV).

In addition, this dissertation is dedicated to my mother, Bessie Taylor Mathis, who inspired me to pursue my dream of helping to ensure that people everywhere are aware of how this disease has affected families throughout the earth; and to my father, Eugene Mathis, who stands behind my endeavors of receiving a quality education.

I wish to dedicate this work to other members of my family who played an instrumental role in shaping my beliefs, character, and integrity: Billy and Flomer Williams, Pinkie and Phillip Bridges, Tom Hearns Jr., Cyprien and Norma Vigilant, and to my sisters: Terrie (in loving memory) Barbara, Shirley, Flora, Denise, and Lakeisha.

I wish to thank my close friends who have encouraged, prayed, and supported me throughout this process: Eric Richard, Jannette Watts, Loretta B. Jones, and Cecelia Ward.

ACKNOWLEDGEMENTS

What makes us special is the signature of God on our lives (Lucado, 2000). I wish to acknowledge my committee: Drs. Alex Kadrie (Mentor), Ronald Black and Mary Jo Brinkman my (Committee Members), for their dedicated support and guidance through the work of completing this dissertation. Thank you for your time and input, as each has made a profound impact on my education.

I would like to acknowledge my learning teams and the School of Academic study, at the University of Phoenix, for their continued support through the years, and for exhibiting the true meaning of teamwork.

I will always be indebted to my parents and great-grandmother Sarah Sherrouse who instilled in me grace, fortitude, a firm belief in God, and an insatiable desire for reading and learning.

In addition, to my family members, uncles, aunts, cousins, friends, students, coworkers, professors, and prayer partners . . . , thank you so much for your encouragement, wisdom, and support. Your contributions were needed and appreciated, and many thanks for believing in me.

And "now unto Him who is able to do exceeding abundantly above all that we ask or think, according to the power that worketh in us, Unto Him be glory . . ." (Ephesians 3:20, 21 KJV).

TABLE OF CONTENTS

LIST OF TABLES

LIST OF FIGURES

CHAPTER 1

INTRODUCTION

In the last decade, the global pandemic of HIV/AIDS has disrupted the lives of millions of people in the United States (Stampley, 2005). HIV disproportionately affects African Americans, as with many other diseases of poverty and limited resources. The spreading of HIV has been influenced by poverty, lack of access to health care, distrust of health systems, inadequate resources, and a myriad of other social factors and inequities (Global Campaign for Microbicides, 2006). Although African Americans only account for 13 percent of the U.S. population, African Americans account for half of all new AIDS diagnoses in the U.S. (Global-Campaign, 2006).

The solution for this type of epidemic is not short-term. Strategists should look 10-30 years ahead for ways to prevent the disease. Prevention may bridge the gap between those who are HIV negative, HIV positive, and/or infected with AIDS (Global AIDS Epidemic, 2005). Almost 40 percent of newly diagnosed HIV positive women in the U.S. are African American (Yellin, 2006), and 23 times more likely to be diagnosed with AIDS than white women (CDC, 2005). The study may inspire a closer review of lack of awareness and their socio-economic status of African American women affected by HIV/AIDS.

Increasing interests have emerged from leader's perspective on HIV/AIDS awareness. This introduction addresses two different audiences. It is both an introduction for persons not familiar with AIDS and the HIV updates, and a resource for activists; it includes information not generally available in one compilation (AIDS. gov, 2010). This chapter provides a theoretical foundation for the remaining chapters. The study examines the purpose of the role of leadership and problems for research on HIV/AIDS awareness and includes a research method, design, and questionnaire to seek awareness results. The results offer a leadership perspective of in-depth awareness and insight about how HIV/AIDS affects African American women.

Background of the Problem

Singer and Baer (2007) report that acquired immune deficiency syndrome (AIDS) has emerged as one of the most devastating diseases in human history. "The virus that causes AIDS, human immunodeficiency virus (HIV), has spread rapidly throughout the world's human population" (Singer & Baer, 2007, p. 201). According to Fauci (2008), Auto-Immunodeficiency Syndrome is the full-blown case of an infection with the Human Immuno Virus I or II, a retrovirus.

According to Smith and Daniel (2006) a retrovirus that causes AIDS by infecting helper T-cells of the immune system was the most common serotype, HIV-1. This retrovirus was distributed worldwide while HIV-2 was primarily confined to West Africa. The disease was termed HIV when the person becomes just infected (Fauci, 2008). The virus has the power of replication, so that the virus remains unharmed by treatment. The HIV virus must infect other cells in order to replicate, and other opportunistic viruses enter the human body, leaving behind the advantage of immunity. The HIV virus will progress, weaken the body cells, and reach its full-fledged state of AIDS.

According to Health Scout Network (2009) immediately following infection with HIV, most individuals develop a brief, nonspecific viral illness consisting of low-grade fever, rash, muscle aches, headache, and/or fatigue. Like any other viral illness, these symptoms resolve over a period of five to ten days. Then for a period of several years (sometimes as long as several decades), people infected with HIV were asymptomatic (no symptoms). Then, the virus gradually destroys their immune system. When this destruction has progressed to a critical point, symptoms of AIDS appear. These symptoms are as follows: extreme fatigue; rapid weight loss from an unknown cause (more than 10 lbs. in two months for no reason); the appearance of swollen or tender glands in the neck, armpits or groin, for no apparent reason, lasting for more than four weeks; unexplained shortness of breath, frequently accompanied by a dry cough, not due to allergies or smoking; persistent diarrhea; intermittent high fever or soaking night sweats of unknown origin; a marked change in an illness pattern, either in frequency, severity, or length of sickness; the appearance of one or more purple spots on the surface of the skin, inside the mouth, anus or nasal passages; whitish coating on the tongue, throat or vagina; and forgetfulness, confusion and other signs of mental deterioration. "It can take as short as a year to as long as 10 to 15 years to go from being infected with HIV to 'full-blown' AIDS" (Health Scout Network, 2009, p. 2).

HIV/AIDS signifies the presence of opportunistic infections, which could affect any part of the body and present as pneumonia (Fauci, 2008). The first case was identified in the United States (U.S.) in homosexuals who presented with pneumonia in 1981. Since 1981, more than 1.6 million people have been infected with HIV/AIDS (CDC, 2004).

Problem Statement

In the Dallas and Fort Worth areas of Texas, we are seeing an increase in the incidence of HIV/AIDS amongst African American women. The increase in the infection population brings additional awareness of this disease to the community but infection rates continue to rise and families continue to suffer losses, when African American women die from this disease. Many issues contribute to the problem of increasing death rates and escalating occurrences of HIV/AIDS among African American women (Census, 2007). The increase in death and infection rates presented an urgent need to develop awareness related to the prevention of HIV/AIDS (Wilson, 2010).

The epidemiology research stated by the CDC (2009) and reported by the AIDS Education Global Information System, supports HIV/AIDS prevention findings about the two cities, Dallas and Fort Worth,

Texas. Each city has received more than $1 million in city funding over the past three years to support HIV/AIDS prevention (CDC, 2009). The HIV/AIDS Prevention Research Synthesis (PRS) project, initiated by the Prevention Research Branch Division of HIV/AIDS Prevention (DHAP) at CDC in 1996, systematically reviews and summarizes HIV behavioral prevention research literature (CDC, 2009). The epidemiological goal of PRS is to translate scientific evidence from the research literature into practical information that is utilizable by prevention providers at state and local health departments throughout the United States and HIV prevention researchers (CDC, 2009). Given this goal, important steps may be taken to conduct more research on the effectiveness of prevention, as measures could relate to HIV/AIDS prevention.

This qualitative grounded theory study explored and identified the level of HIV/AIDS awareness in African American women in the Dallas and Fort Worth areas of Texas. This research study used a population sample of 30 African American women. The study used several data collection methods, such as observations, interviews, and questionnaires to report the findings on HIV/AIDS awareness. The results are presented as an informational tool about HIV/AIDS awareness, which may increase effective prevention of HIV/AIDS.

Purpose of the Study

The purpose of this qualitative grounded theory research study was to explore HIV/AIDS awareness in African American women from the Dallas and Fort Worth areas of Texas. Quantification was not possible in the present situation therefore the intention was to elicit subjective information from the participants. Many aspects of African American women's knowledge pertaining to this disease were unearthed from the participants via a HIV/AIDS awareness questionnaire. The strategy for this research design was to inform African American women in Dallas and Fort Worth, Texas, about the impact of the HIV/AIDS disease. The primary value of this current study lies in the questionnaire results possibly leading to increased HIV/AIDS prevention and awareness. Additional benefits also lie in finding opportunities to connect the study to existing theoretical formulations obtained from participants at community colleges in Dallas and Fort Worth, Texas.

Significance of the Study

The significance of this current study is the number of women with HIV (human immunodeficiency virus) infection and AIDS (acquired immunodeficiency syndrome) has increased steadily worldwide. According to the World Health Organization (WHO), by the end of 2005, 17.5 million women worldwide were infected with HIV (National Institutes of Health—NIH, 2007 & Fauci, 2009). Efforts to promote responsible awareness and accountability in the community with churches have placed attention on the fact that African American women are dying of the infection of HIV/AIDS (Centers for Disease Control and Prevention, 2008).

The results method and design are useful to the City of Dallas and the City of Fort Worth, Texas. The newspapers in these cities could inform the community about the implications and raise their levels of awareness. The possible benefits of such reports could encourage more cities and community leaders to get involved in HIV/AIDS awareness.

Significance to the Study of Leadership

In the 1990s, the federal AIDS care budget failed to keep pace with the epidemic (Gerald & Wright, 2008). Community leaders have seriously challenged the Dallas and Fort Worth areas of Texas, with prevention and management incidences (Bryant, 2009). The involvement of leaders in the community has improved awareness and brought about indifference from those affected by HIV/AIDS (Bryant, 2009).

The HIV/AIDS epidemic is having an increasingly disproportionate impact on African American leaders, who represent those already disadvantaged populations: African American women (Kaiser Family Foundation, 1998). AIDS is spreading throughout the African American community closing the gap on those who are not infected (Biology News, 2006). The U.S. Department of Health and Human Services (2009) reports the results of increased awareness have become an informational tool to inform and possibly prevent the spread of HIV/AIDS.

Nature of the Study

Kaiser Family Foundation (1998) reports showed that HIV/AIDS results are representative of African American women nationwide. The nature of this current study represented African American women in Dallas and Fort Worth, Texas. The results provided new perspectives and insights regarding African American women's awareness of the HIV/AIDS disease. Much of the research contributed to an increased awareness about the ways in which social and cultural contexts shape women's knowledge of HIV/AIDS. The existing literature on African American women's awareness levels suggests HIV/AIDS has seriously challenged our nation calling into question many of our approaches to understanding diseases, prevention, treatment, and management (Kaiser Family Foundation, 1998, p.1).

Research Method

A use of qualitative research uses open-ended techniques such as interviews to collect data for understanding issues or human behavior in terms of reasons for the behavior and elicits the understandings and motives, which cause some actions (Clissett, 2008). This sampling illustrated results from 30 African American women in the Dallas and Fort Worth area. The participants are not a representative group but they were expected to provide some knowledge about the lack of awareness of HIV/AIDS in the African American population (Tavakol, 2006). In quantitative research, the relationships between two individual or two sets of variables are compared: The independent variable and the dependent variables are usually the outcome. They aim to "study things in their natural setting, attempting to make sense of, interpret, and realize phenomena in terms of the meanings people bring to them, and they use 'a holistic perspective', which preserves the complexities of human behavior" (Greenhalgh & Taylor, 2008, p.1).

Quantitative research did not serve this current study's purpose. Quantitative research deals with numerical data. For an accurate estimation of the relationship between the variables in a descriptive quantitative research, hundreds of participants may be required. The large number was not possible here; the costs would multiply to impossible limits. The variables were not identified; therefore, a quantitative descriptive research was not appropriate.

In the experimental quantitative research, subjects are measured before and/or after a treatment. Treatment or any interventions were not involved in the present study. The experimental quantitative research was not applicable here (Creswell, 2002). Future study could be done using the experimental quantitative method of research using the basic ideas obtained from this qualitative study, followed by interventions to increase awareness and then reassessing the awareness. A control group without interventions could also be instituted and studied for comparison. The mixed variety of research employs a quantitative and qualitative research. This was not required as the objective was to elicit maximum unknown information from a selected sample of African American women in a particular area.

Research Design

The grounded theory design was employed for this current study using a qualitative approach. The foundation of grounded theory evolved from Symbolic Interactionism where human beings are seen as the key participants and shapers of this world (Coleman & O'Connor, 2007). The theory was first established by Glaser and Strauss (1967) having been derived from the constant comparative method. This study started with few predetermined ideas and increased in depth of awareness. Towards the end of the study, a set of relationships were evolved that had a systematic theoretical framework and explained relevant social, psychological and/or educational, or events of awareness (Coleman & O'Connor, 2007). A theory evolved from continuous interplay between data collection and analysis. Good theory development was insured by the process of breaking down interviews, observations, and other forms of appropriate data into distinct units of meaning, which are labeled to generate concepts (Coleman & O'Connor, 2007).

The grounded theory method was the right design to incorporate in this research. The theoretical sampling was completed first.

The 30 African American women of the Dallas/Fort Worth areas were distributed questionnaires about lack of awareness of HIV/AIDS. The questions in the first few samples were changed as the interviewer continued with the addition of new questions as new ideas were gathered from the first few answers. Noticing an emergent category, the questions were reframed to benefit the category. This became an ever-changing process and constant comparison was evident. The data collection framed the study, as the information was gathered from the participants. An awareness theory was developed throughout the study. The research questions were changed to benefit new requirements. The nature of data analysis was inductive and interpretive. Through selective sampling, saturation of categories, research variables emerged from the study. Then characteristics of the core variable were repeated. The results linked and explained various data, and had implications for a general or formal theoretical theory, and helped to study maximum variations and analysis.

The results from the questionnaires were analyzed line-by-line using NVIVO coding processes. These results were recorded from the participants' answers, and are not the interpretations of the researcher. Many levels of codes were made following each set of interviews (Coleman & O'Connor, 2007). The main categories were divided into subcategories, which are known as axial coding. Selective coding is a process of re-integrating and redefining of the theory. The core category was then identified. Formal communication was the process of making notes and ideas from the information. These communication strategies were used in the form of questions and statements. They are the building blocks of the final theory (Coleman & O'Connor, 2007). The process involved in reaching the theory was gradual and progressive. The participants' answers were collected and recorded. Attempts were made to categorize the answers. Then the answers were coded based on the results. Redefining and reassessing the codes were completed and theories were formed with particular relevance to the lack of awareness of HIV/AIDS.

Research Questions

All research is socially constructed (Martin, 2007). Two research questions guided the study:

RQ1. What are adverse implications of African American women acquiring HIV/AIDS after awareness measures have been in place?

RQ2. What do African American women know about the impact of the HIV/AIDS epidemic?

Theoretical Framework

The study results revealed many facts relating to the behaviors of African American women. Emphasis was placed on the women of the Dallas and Fort Worth communities, who are silent sufferers. The theoretical framework of these interventions created a superlative interest in light of the community and enlightening awareness that a gap in awareness does exists throughout the nation (Centers for Disease Control and Prevention, 2008). The application of social constructionist theory to literacy's community context reflects the important social forces framing the changes in awareness in 2003 (Leu, Kinzer, Coiro, & Cammack, 2004). The results from the policies have shown that targeting of specific populations produces the maximum positive and cost-effective results.

Baleta (2004) report that both programs (behavioral and awareness) are intended to be successful in the community. The programs appear to be better than preventive initiatives on a large scale where the emphasis is on informing more women about HIV/AIDS than introducing prevention measures on a smaller scale. The benefits from the scope of the study revealed that repetition of meeting with the same persons gained interest in awareness about HIV/AIDS for reinforcing the important messages (Baleta, 2004).

African American women were selected for this research. The women represent those affected with HIV/AIDS in Dallas and Fort Worth, Texas. The Centers for Disease Control and Prevention (2005) report that these two areas encompass 49 percent of African American women infected, when their population forms just 13 percent of the all total HIV/AIDS cases in the Dallas and Fort Worth areas as shown in Figure 1 (HIV/AIDS Factsheet, 2005). This figure demonstrates that approximately half (49 percent) of those diagnosed with HIV/AIDS in 2005 were black (according to information from 33 states).

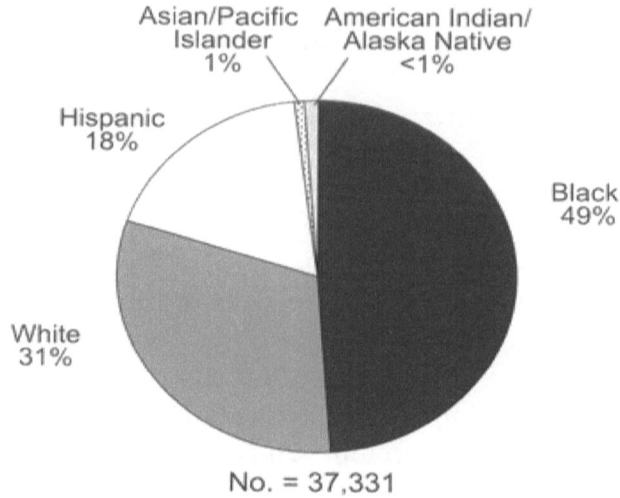

No. = 37,331

Figure 1. About Half (49 percent) of People Infected are Black/Racial Breakdown/2005.

Castro and Farmer (2005) revealed that a theoretical framework for the understanding of HIV/AIDS related awareness has been developed over a decade of ethnographic research. An interpretation of the relevant information was informed by more recent illustrations providing social theories (Farmer & Kleinman, 1989). Although the first references to the association between shame and health in the social science literature date back to the 1880s, sociologist have developed what has become the benchmark social theory of the association between stigma and disease. Goffman (1961) defines stigma as the identification that a social group creates of a person (or group of people) based on some physical, behavioral, or social trait perceived as being divergent from group norms. Goffman (1961) notes this socially constructed theory lays the groundwork, for subsequent disqualification of membership from a group in which that person was originally included. Although he emphasized the importance of analyzing stigma in terms of relationships rather than individual traits or attributes, many subsequent interpretations of stigma have focused on individual attributes and are separate from broader social processes, especially from relations of social power (1963).

Definitions and Abbreviations

African American

An American, who is black and has lived in U.S.A., or Canada following transatlantic settlement. Generally, African Americans, also known as black Americans have family characteristics, such as strong kinship bonds, strong work orientation, adaptable family roles, high achievement orientation, and strong religious orientation (Hairston & Smith, 1983).

Acyclovir

A nucleoside analog antiviral drug used to treat the symptoms of herpes simplex virus infection, herpes zoster (shingles), and sometimes-acute varicella zoster virus (chicken pox) (Hovanesian, 2008).

Advancing HIV Prevention—AHP

Its aim is to reduce barriers to early diagnosis of HIV infection and increase access to quality medical care, treatment, and ongoing prevention services for HIV-positive persons and their partners. The AHP initiative represents a multi-agency collaboration within the (Department of Health and Human Services, 2003).

Acquired Immune Deficiency Syndrome—AIDS

A diagnosis of AIDS is made whenever a person is HIV-positive and he or she has a CD4+ cell count below 200 cells per micro liter or his or her CD4+ cells account for fewer than 14 percent of all lymphocytes or that person has been diagnosed with one or more of the AIDS-defining diseases (Peters, 2008).

CD4/T Cells—CD4 Cells

On its surface, these cells have molecules called CD4. These helper cells initiate the body's response to invading microorganisms such as viruses. T-cells are specialized white blood cells that play an important role in the body's immune system (Malviya, Hasan, & Hussain, 2009).

Down Low

The most generic definition of the term down low, or DL, is to keep something private, whether information or activity. The term is often used to describe the behavior of men who have intimate relationships with other men as well as women and who do not identify as gay or bisexual. These men may refer to themselves as being "on the down low," "on the DL," or "on the low." The term has most often been associated with African American men. Although the term originated in the African American community, the behaviors associated with the term are not new and not specific to black men who have intimate relationships with men. Beyond the Down Low," focuses on the underground subculture of men who have sex with men, and who project a heterosexual public image (Boykin, 2005).

HAART

Highly active anti-retroviral therapy, analyzes the effects of an intrapartum dose of nevirapine to prevent mother-to-child HIV transmission (Harding, Molloy, Easterbrook, Frame, & Higginson, 2006).

HIV

Human Immunodeficiency Virus is a retrovirus that causes AIDS by infecting helper T cells of the immune system (American Heritage Dictionary, 2000).

IDU

Injection Drug Users (Tarakeshwar, Kalichman, Simbayi, & Sikkema, 2008).

Minority HIV/AIDS research initiative—MARI

Community Education Groups (CEG) understands the importance of research in the development of viable programs and policies that reflect the needs and concerns of the communities they are designed to help. With this understanding, CEG has been striven to develop a research program that examines the issues of Black women, their families and communities as expressed from the African American communities affected and infected by this disease (Centers for Disease Control and Prevention, 2007).

Needle Exchange Program—NEP

Needle-exchange programs, or NEPs, are community-based initiatives that allow intravenous (IV) drug users to exchange used syringes for clean, sterile ones in an effort to stem the spread of HIV/ AIDS, hepatitis B and other blood-borne pathogens. NEPs generally provide HIV/AIDS education, testing and condoms, as well as abuse treatment referrals (Tarakeshwar, Kalichman, Simbayi, & Sikkema, 2008).

Prevention of Mother to Child Transmission—PMTCT

A committee organized by the Center for Disease Control and Prevention to monitor and decrease HIV transmission from women infected with HIV to their infants (Tarakeshwar, Kalichman, Simbayi, & Sikkema, 2008).

Post Exposure Prophylaxis—PEP

PEP is just what the name suggests; prophylaxis (preventative) medications given after an HIV or suspected HIV exposure in hopes of decreasing the likelihood of HIV infection from the exposure. The PEP medication combinations used depends on the degree of exposure and the HIV status of the source of the exposure. Before any medications are prescribed, it has to be determined if PEP is indicated and appropriate (Gritzmacher, Cody, Minick, & Sowell, 2007).

Retrovirus

In 1977, earlier retravirus (1974), from re(verse) tra(nscriptase) + virus. The virus is called a retravirus because it contains reverse transcriptase, an enzyme that uses RNA instead of DNA to encode genetic information, which reverses the usual pattern. This is remodeled by inflammation of retro-backwards (Smith & Daniel, 2006).

Sisters Informing Sisters on Topics about AIDS—SISTA

A group-level, social skills training intervention for African American women aimed at reducing HIV intimate risk behaviors (Collins, Whiters, & Braithwaite, 2007).

National Association of People Living with AIDS—NAPWA

Established to convince those with HIV to announce their status (Baleta, 2004).

Women Involved in Life Learning from Other Women—WILLOW

WILLOW brings together women of different ages, races, and religious backgrounds with the common bond of being women faced with a similar challenge, while managing LIFE around HIV (Wingood & DiClemente, 2006).

Assumptions

According to Merriam (1998), "the key philosophical assumption . . . upon which all types of qualitative research are based, is the view that reality is constructed by individuals interacting with their social worlds" (p. 20). Merriam (1988, 1998) and Creswell (1994) outline several additional underlying assumptions and characteristics of qualitative research:

1. Qualitative researchers are interested in understanding the meaning people have constructed.

2. Reality is holistic, multidimensional, and ever changing; it is not a single, fixed, objective phenomenon waiting to be discovered, observed, and measured as in quantitative research.
3. The researcher is the primary instrument for data collection and analysis.
4. Qualitative research usually involves fieldwork.
5. Qualitative research primarily employs an inductive research strategy.
6. Qualitative research focuses on process.
7. The product of a qualitative study is richly descriptive.
8. The design of a qualitative study is emergent and flexible (Merriam, 1998).

The assumption was that HIV/AIDS information is suited for those who do not have HIV/AIDS. The research provided key information about prevention. Adults, between the ages of 18 and 54 are more sexually active. This age group should be cautious and develop attitudes and behavioral patterns that supports prevention, as this group has an opportunity to become exposed to the HIV/AIDS disease (UNAIDS, 1997). In spite of the important role of public representatives in the world, the bulk of information about HIV/AIDS has been focused on those already infected by the disease. Few studies focus on prevention of those in this age group (UNAIDS, 1997). In general, public representatives have an implicit assumption that, when given the correct information, a reduction in HIV/AIDS in the African American communities may be reduced over time (UNAIDS, 1997).

Scope of the Study

The purpose of this qualitative, grounded theory research presented evidence on HIV/AIDS awareness and the scope of this study encompassed thirty African American women in the Dallas and Fort Worth areas of Texas. Surveys were provided by random selection to uncover the level of awareness; or to identify prevention measures against HIV/AIDS.

Limitations

This research has several limitations. First, because of the sensitive nature of the questionnaires, findings are subject to social desirability bias. Second, there was the possibility of inducing bias since participants were expected to provide information on previous intimate behaviors. The cities where the participating college students came from were predetermined, and not all the participants responded to all survey questions. The participants who did not answer all of the questions might be different in their sexual behaviors from those who answered all questions. Finally, because of the small sample size and the fact that some college students had college degrees and others did not possess a college degree at the time of the surveys, might pose a limitation. A study with a larger sample involving more participants would provide more information.

In spite of the stated limitations, the findings from this research have several implications for the design and implementation of HIV/AIDS prevention interventions on college campuses in Dallas and Fort Worth, Texas. It was obvious that a "one size fits all" approach of disseminating research information could not be taken with this research (Adefuye, Abiona, Balogun, & Durrel, 2009). The low rates of African American women with knowledge about HIV/AIDS awareness may be due to poor negotiating skills, poor health care uses of self-worth or apathy to the HIV/AIDS epidemic; a combination of these factors need further study (Adefuye, Abiona, Balogun, & Durrel, 2009). Alcohol and drugs use were not a major factor in the participants of this research. It is therefore important that HIV/AIDS prevention interventions for African American women in Dallas and Fort Worth, Texas, incorporate drug and alcohol education, particularly in the context of intimate activity in research.

Delimitations

There were two components to comprise the focus of this study. The first component consisted of thirty African American women from the cities of Dallas and Fort Worth Texas. The second component consisted of questionnaires to elicit the women's level of awareness with regard to HIV/AIDS, and other women were not considered.

This current study was delimited to African American women in two major cities in Texas. All other races, with the exception of African American women were not included in this sample to prevent skewing of the results. Women who do not meet the study criteria were excluded from this study.

Summary

This chapter presented an overview of the proposed study to examine HIV/AIDS awareness, perceptions, and behavior practices among African American women in the Dallas and Fort Worth areas of Texas (Haynes, Chng, & Vosvick, 2008). Finally, this study examined perceptions of HIV/AIDS threat and attitudes towards one's motivation to participate in personal and public awareness, and prevention measures that assisted in awareness and prevention of the HIV/AIDS disease among African American women (Hill & Vosvick, 2008). Based on a theoretical framework illustrating the information, a grounded theory research design was employed for this study using a qualitative approach to assess the study theories. The questionnaire instrument developed and utilized was Qualitative Data Collection: ethnographic participant observation, and unstructured interviews (Newman, 2002).

Chapter 2 presents a review of literature related to HIV/AIDS awareness, past research about awareness, and subsequent prevention. The illustration of literature traces the history of local, state, national, and federal information and prevention in relation to HIV/AIDS awareness. Highlighted is literature from community and federal awareness representatives, which addresses African American women and HIV/AIDS.

CHAPTER 2

LITERATURE REVIEW

The purpose of this current study was to examine African American women's awareness of HIV/AIDS. The Auto Immune Deficiency Syndrome or AIDS have spread globally resulting in a pandemic. There are 33.2 million people affected by HIV/AIDS, and the national range is 30.6 to 36.1 million in 2007, (WHO, 2007). A reduction was evident from the previous year's estimate of 39.5 million (UNAIDS, 2006).

One reason for the difference was attributed to the correction of India's contribution to the figure. New estimates also differed in that HIV infections and deaths were obtained by considering prevalence estimates, new incidences, and mortality in 2007. The actual figures were not affected at all (WHO, 2007). Refinements in methodology are one of the main reasons for different or reduced figures.

The literature within Chapter 2 provides a review of the literature concerning the shock of the HIV/AIDS pandemic on African American women; women of all races, and an overview of HIV/AIDS in African American communities in Dallas and Fort Worth, Texas. The study was based on a theoretical framework upon which was detailed, with the development of the study questionnaire instrument; the qualitative grounded theory approach, which is explained later in this chapter.

Historical Overview

Historically, in order to go back to the origin of the problem, the Literature Review encompasses data from 1967 to 2010, in order to cover the private and public, local, state, and national awareness issues about African American women and HIV/AIDS. The literature review was useful to illustrate the historical aspect of informing the participants about HIV/AIDS awareness. In effect, the historical data benefits women of all races, in that the data improves awareness about the HIV/AIDS disease and reduce the death rate of women dying with this terrible disease.

The first instances of HIV infection were believed to have come from the chimpanzees and sooty mangabey monkeys in Africa (Gao, Bailes, Robertson, & Chen, 1999). Transmission of infected virus occurs through sexual contact with an infected partner and by sharing contaminated injection equipment (Gao et al., 1999). Prior to screening procedures, blood transfusions are another mode of transmission. Accidental needle pricks in the health care setting do not usually cause transmission due to post exposure prophylaxis.

The CD4+ cells of the immune system helps the body to fight disease by responding to any infection. HIV damages these cells when the body becomes infected, and thereby weakens the ability of the body to fight disease. HIV causes the body to be prone to opportunistic infections such as syphilis, tuberculosis, protozoal, and fungal infections similar to pneumocystitis, carinii, and pneumonia; malignancies such as Kaposi's sarcoma and lymphoma, viral infections, as Herpes simplex, cytomegalovirus and neurological conditions of AIDS dementia complex (Gao, et al., 1999).

Title Searches, Articles, Research Documents, and Journals

An abundance of information and research literature is available in the areas of HIV/AIDS awareness, and preventive measures. No research studies address correlation between awareness and prevention in the Dallas and Fort Worth areas of Texas. The literature review illustrates key terms and abbreviations associated with HIV/AIDS awareness and preventions, and awareness among African American women.

Anti-Retroviral Treatment

Treatment is classified into the protease inhibitors, nucleoside analog reverse transcriptase inhibitors (NRTIs), and non-nucleoside analog reverse transcriptase inhibitors (NNRTs). The protease inhibitors interfere with the HIV assembling and release from the CD4+ cells. The NRTIs incorporate into the genetic material of the virus and prevent its building up. The NNRTs bind with the reverse transcriptase and prevent the duplication of viral genetic materials (National Institutes of Allergy and Infectious Diseases, 2002). Combination therapies from all the classes help prevent drug resistance. Despite cost reductions and increased availability, poor countries cannot afford the costly anti-retroviral therapy or do not have access to them. The HAART is the new standard method of medical treatment.

Prevention Objectives

The main objective about awareness was to reduce HIV incidences that are the number of new cases per year in a population as this would be the main contributor to total existing cases in the population. The more the number of persons living with HIV, the more the chances of progression, the more the risks of transmission and the more the number of resulting deaths (WHO, 2007). The HIV/AIDS prevention research has shown that interventions that target risk behaviors, improve knowledge are committed to awareness and disease prevention. The prevention relates to one or more of the priority areas that the Planning Grants for HIV/AIDS Prevention and Treatment agency would investigate in 2010 (Ory, 2001).

Preventive Techniques Employed Earlier

The historical evidence and prevention strategies dealt with voluntary counseling and testing that reduced the incidence of unprotected sex. Only those who came forward benefited (Tarakeshwar et al., 2008). Then the promotion of condom use especially in relationship to sex workers was introduced as an awareness and prevention tool. The prevention was strictly enforced in places approximating Thailand where the principle of "No condom, no sex" was followed (Tarakeshwar et al., 2008). The disadvantage is the process worked well only where sex workers were organized. Prevention of mother-to-child transmission (PMTCT) program provided counseling, testing, and treatment. The stigma of poor infrastructure and difficult access restricts the benefits of this method (Tarakeshwar et al., 2008). Even influential sex workers had been selected to be peers in places like Calcutta, India. The representatives in India found that 25 percent of the incidence of AIDS increased, when consistent use was observed compared to 15 percent decrease in the control community, while the general use (inconsistent) increased by 39 percent and in the control community by 11 percent (Basu et al., 2004).

Sexually transmitted infections (STI's) screening and treatment was another effective prevention strategy. The success of this program varied in different nations. Tanzania and Thailand indicated a decrease in the STI's including AIDS (Tarakeshwar et al., 2008). Alcohol prevention programs, alcohol rehabilitation programs, needle exchange programs were some of the programs targeted at youths in order to reduce their high-risk behavior about HIV. The success of these programs is on an increase. The needle exchange program was successful in Brazil and developed countries (Tarakeshwar, 2008). HIV prevention for homosexual men had reduced the incidence of unprotected anal sex and decreased the number of partners. In India it was difficult to measure success as many gender identities existed and stigma had made many of the men with altered identity marry according to their family wishes (Tarakeshwar et al., 2008). There were 22 school based sex and HIV prevention programs in developing countries that can reduce risky behaviors by delaying the sexual activity, reducing the frequency of the act, decreasing the number of partners, increasing the use of condoms and reducing unprotected sex (Kirby, Obasi, & Laris, 2006). Only 13 of the 22 programs could be merited to meeting rigorous implementation standards.

More Innovative Techniques for Prevention

Tarakeshwar (2008) reports that none of the above-mentioned methods were considered fool proof protection. An interdisciplinary approach combining biomedical, social and behavioral sciences should be considered for future HIV prevention. Prevention programs including "male circumcision, microbicides, cervical barriers, herpes suppression, antiretroviral treatment (ART) to prevent sexual transmission, and HIV vaccines" are in the late stage of trials (Tarakeshwar, 2008, p. 19). These methods were combined with approaches prevalent now and in the future, when dealing with the behavioral changes of the people at risk. The male circumcision could be combined with HIV testing and counseling services, STI treatment, promotion of safer intimate practices, provision and promotion of consistent use of the male and female condoms (WHO, 2007). Research resulted about determining whether Acyclovir reduced HIV transmission. Acyclovir was used to prevent Herpes simplex, an STI that increases the risk of HIV acquisition and transmission (Bertozzi et al., 2006). Female controlled or initiated methods like microbicides and cervical barrier methods were strongly considered for promotion. The promotion helped to reduce the infection in women. HIV vaccines were considered the long-term hope for prevention (Tarakeshwar et al., 2008).

Policy interventions addressing "gender inequality, education, housing, nutritional resources, economic opportunities like microfinance, access to credit and property rights" were evaluated at the population level (Tarakeshwar et al., 2008, p. 20). In regards to substance abuse, two opioid agonist medications, methadone and buprenorphine, effectively treat dependence on opioids (Tilson et al., 2006). The relevance of mental health in HIV transmission was studied. Newer strategies that were discussed globally are the Provider Initiated Testing and counseling. All patients who came to the health clinic were counseled and tested routinely, for HIV.

Advantages of Newer Interventions

Crepaz (2006) posits that prevention techniques were targeted to small populations that were at risk for HIV/AIDS. Interventions aimed at these specific groups with specific behaviors and diverse problems appear to produce better results. Large-scale prevention strategies could only pass on messages resulting in larger numbers to reach the infected persons, but with no assurance, the messages had touched them or changed the existing behaviors. Recent studies are concentrating on smaller pockets of positively infected persons with their partners and women visiting incarcerated men (Crepaz, 2006).

Prevention among HIV Infected Population

The first interventions followed the Social Cognitive theory based on the principles of behavior change. Risk reduction was evident when counseling in small groups and individually (Crepaz et al., 2006). Interventions combined with skill building produced better results. Longer duration interventions are better accepted than the short ones but those related to ongoing services are not so productive. The second intervention was the prevention approaches for the HIV infected would imply smaller and more definite numbers are involved. Frequent and consistent approaches would definitely change their transmission rate to unsuspecting partners (Tarakeshwar et al., 2008). Simply disclosing the fact that he or she was infected can reduce transmission by 40 percent (Tarakeshwar et al., 2008). The program among the targeted HIV infected also turns out to be more effective and cost-effective (Tarakeshwar et al., 2008). Only, one-third of the infected people continue with high-risk behaviors (Tarakeshwar et al., 2008). The CDC has made prevention plans for infected people a high-priority, naming it "Prevention for Positives." This policy has been adopted in developing countries such as India (Tarakeshwar et al., 2008).

National Association of People Living with AIDS (NAPWA)

NAPWA represents National Association of People living with AIDS. A cost saving strategy was postulated by a study in a California University based clinic (Baleta, 2004). The objective was to prevent at-risk people living with HIV/AIDS, from transmission of infection to uninfected sexual or injection drug-using partners. This idea helped to reduce the expenditure to be afforded on the at-risk populations thereby decreasing the disease burden too (Copenhaver & Fisher, 2006). The most effective strategy reduced the rate of new infections through improved targeting of prevention messages (Copenhaver

& Fisher, 2006). The medical setting was found as the best place for promoting prevention messages. Screening for risk behaviors, communicating preventive messages that have a better chance of reinforcing safe behavior, referring patients for substance abuse treatment, making easy partner notification, counseling with leaders, who are seen as respectful, caring, and committed to community involvement, testing and identifying other STI are facilitated at the medical clinic (Baleta, 2004). A theory-driven behavioral approach provided in a clinical setting contributed to effective prevention strategies being developed (Trochim, 2006). The Prevention with Positives idea was followed in the study named NAPWA conducted by the NAPWA association in 2004.

Women Cohabiting with Incarcerated Men

Incarceration or imprisonment was one opportunity that was listed in the spread of the HIV/AIDS (Grinstead, 2008). Preventive interventions were planned just for the prisoners and the family member of the prisoners. Low rates of condom use, hardly any HIV testing done and the lack of awareness of prison-related risks of HIV all play a role in the spread of disease among the group of women and incarcerated partners. Peer education could transform behaviors of the at-risk group. Intervention programs are flexible and conforming to the sentiments of the population at risk (Grinstead, 2008).

The world's highest incarceration rate was indentified in the U.S. (Grinstead, 2008). The large population of 2.2 million jailed men constitutes a mobile population that moves toward the families, usually in the low-income group and in the African American community. Thus, correctional confinement or incarceration contributes to an impact on public health. The prevalence of confirmed AIDS cases among the prisoners was 3.5 times the incidence in the general population in 2004. The AIDS cases are 0.5 percent as against 0.1 5 percent (Grinstead, 2008). The incidence was higher considering that not all prisoners took an AIDS test. Educational interventions with peers, peer-led interventions for pre-release prisoners, health promotion interventions for HIV seropositive pre-release prisoners and hepatitis prevention interventions are implemented for pre-release prisoners (Grinstead, 2008).

According to the wishes of the prisoners, interventions for their wives were planned. The women who were African American and low income had high rates of infections similar to the prisoners. Grinstead (2008) reports 80 percent of infections were caused by unprotected sex with a seropositive man. The chance of having a partner who was incarcerated increased the risk of infection (Grinstead, 2008). In addition, Grinstead (2008) reports 50 percent of prisoners claim to have a female partner waiting for them, once released from prison. Interventions prevalent now do not focus on whether the women have a previously incarcerated partner (Grinstead, 2008). Literature has revealed that interventions need to address gender differences, to utilize the services of peers and have multiple sessions to make a better impact. The interventions also needed to be acceptable to the population. The women who were visiting incarcerated men had time constraints, could hardly make themselves available, are not inclined to wait around after visiting and usually have small children with them at the time of the visit. The women were also fearful of making disclosures, which could harm their men in prison (Grinstead, 2008). An added factor about HIV was not the primary concern now of visiting incarcerated men. The concerns were those of healthcare for the children, prison visits, parole policies, how to access resources for food, housing, and childcare.

The Health Options Mean Empowerment or (HOME) was planned for the women who are visiting incarcerated men. This intervention concentrates on the women's lives away from prison. Due to the neutral attitude taken by the authorities who implemented the intervention, the women shed inhibitions and participated in the intervention programs (Grinstead, 2008). The entire family of women is encouraged to participate along with the targeted women, who visit the prisons. The idea was to solicit social support for the unfortunate women. Popular interventions are repeated and peer educators have an important role in this program. The women participants who spoke highly of them appreciated the impact. The non-judgmental approach helped the women become more relaxed about the interventions. The women are also introduced to support services in their areas, as the programs are cost effective and would benefit everyone in the end.

Funding Interventions

Increased funding for the various preventive measures and investments in HIV interventions, treatment, and care accounted for the decline of new cases and the longevity of HIV cases. The funding outcomes to Health Departments and HIV Prevention Programs by Source $581,336,729 funding from State, CDC funding $337,006,029, and 7 percent funding from other funding sources $39,065,060 are illustrated in Figure 2.

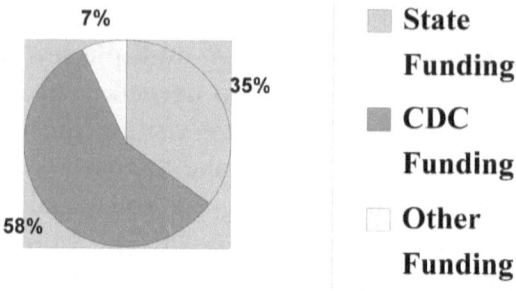

Figure 2. Total FY 2007 HIV Prevention Funding. This figure shows that more than half of this funding came from the CDC. Adapted from: http://www.kff.org/hivaids/upload/7029-03.pdf

The impact of specific measures or interventions that are studied, and may have varied according to the population involved. Studies in specific populations, direct assessments of incidence, mortality, effectiveness of programs, and a detailed study of the problem with women and men have been illustrated. Discovering finite causative details of the incidence was the real reasons for prevalence in certain communities and among African American women would reinforce our knowledge. Even by present standards, the knowledge on HIV/AIDS was far better than any other global disease (WHO, 2007).

Behavioral Theories for HIV Prevention

Serafimovska, Maxwell, and Roberts (2007) report that while the majority of respondents were familiar with the different behavioral theories, 35 percent said they were unfamiliar with Ecological Systems Theories and Social Capital Theory, and about a quarter were not familiar with Diffusion of Innovation Theories, Theories of Gender and Power, and Theories of Reasoned Action (Serafimovska, Maxwell, & Roberts, 2007). About 20 percent were not familiar with Afro Centric Theory, Theory of Individual and Social Change/Empowerment Model, Social Network Theory, Social Cognitive Theory and the Health Belief Model. Only 10 percent were unfamiliar with Stages of Change and the AIDS Risk Reduction Model (Serafimovska, Maxwell, & Roberts, 2007). HIV preventive methods were based on strategies that change people's behaviors, which had the tendency to expose them to risk (Gao et al., 1999). The need to discover behaviors that increase risk of infection through sexual contact and injection drug use were the reasons for devising strategies to change those behaviors, and form the essence of planning interventions. Theory based behavioral interventions form the most contributions of behavioral and social sciences to HIV/AIDS prevention.

Some groups continue to carry medically inaccurate beliefs and baseless opinions. Research has found that there are still people (40 percent) who believe they are prone to infection from a used glass or being coughed or sneezed upon by an infected person (Herek, 2001). Casey (2006) reports that 19 percent of the women interviewed believe those who acquired HIV through sex or drug injection deserved to get the disease. Stigmatizing beliefs were obtained from European Americans who are above 55 years of age, those who had only a high school education, those with a low annual income of less than $30,000, and those with a poorer health status (Gao et al., 1999). Mere factual corrections were insufficient, and sophisticated behavioral theories were monitored, before the interventions were employed in the communities.

Health Belief Model

This model was used during a normal health screening. Health behaviors were believed to be influenced by perceived threat, benefits, barriers, cues to action, self-efficacy, demographics, and other factors that help shape their health beliefs and behaviors (Gao et al., 1999). Perceived threat refers to the person's understanding of how susceptible one can be, with the chance of infection and whether one understands the medical and social consequences. The perceived benefits refer to whether a person who believes the strategies, and would use the knowledge to reduce their threats. The perceived barriers were the fears or negative consequences that would occur if one would try the risk reduction strategies. Cues are the awareness of bodily symptoms, as listed above, or environmental features, which stimulate them into action. Self-efficacy is the degree to which a person believes that he can do a health-related action (Gao et al., 1999). The HIV risk reduction interventions are based on the health belief model, which increased the perceived threats, convince the participants about the efficacy of the strategies planned, and help to find ways to overcome the barriers they expect, enhance their level of awareness and conduct exercises to help them build skills for intervention strategies (Gao et al., 1999).

Theory of Reasoned Action (TRA)

There were several key components mentioned in this section. Behaviors of interests describe four components: target, context, time, and action. One example: females sex workers (targets) in the nearby cities (context) may frequently (time) request their clients permission to use a female condom (action). Prior intention to perform a behavior is the strongest predictor of the actual behavior (Gao et al., 1999). There were two sets of factors which affect strength of intention: individual attitudes and perceived norms. Individual attitudes include the positive and negative attitudes regarding the outcomes of performing the behavior and evaluation of the consequences possible. The perceived norms refer to beliefs about the opinions of others and specific behaviors (e.g., using a condom is safe). Prevention interventions guided by the TRA may promote one or more risk-reduction behaviors after explaining to the person about the pros and cons about the change in behavior and allowing them to see other people in the same or similar condition, who have favorable attitudes towards the specified behavior.

Transtheoretical Model of Change

People are believed to change their behaviors over a period of time, while encountering different stages of life. In the first stage of pre-contemplation, the person would recognize the problem and would not plan any change in behavior. One example: A person does not realize that his relationship with his fiancée, who has had partners before him, may be risky, as he believes that a heterosexual contact cannot cause a risk (Gao et al., 1999). In the contemplative stage, he realizes that he can have a problem out of the relationship and weighs the pros and cons of using a condom. In the third stage or preparation for action, he or she starts using a condom but is inconsistent as he or she may tend to forget the prevention measures. After a few months in the third stage, he or she reaches the fourth stage of action; and, he or she has successfully changed his or her behavior, as becoming consistent in using condoms in his relationship. The final stage of maintenance was reached when he or she has successfully maintained this new behavior for at least six months. People have a habit of oscillating between stages (Prochaska, Norcross, & DiClemente, 1992). This would not be a good practice, because the HIV prevention was not being evaluated. The person administering or monitoring the interventions must work; so that the person he or she was assessing could return to the stage they were initially, to ensure progression onto the next stage was successful through the appropriate interventions. The attention to prevention and interventions become individualistic in nature (Prochaska, Norcross, & DiClemente, 1994).

The Diffusion of Innovations Theory

This theory suggests, "Innovations pass through communication channels among members of a society over time" (Gao et al., 1999). The first stage of knowledge allowed the person to become familiar with new knowledge or existence of a new innovation. In the next stage of persuasion, he or she was motivated to use the innovation by a friend or social worker. In the stage of decision, he or she decides to use the innovation and conforms to the new changes. In the fourth stage of implementation, he or she started to change behaviors. In the stage of reinforcement, he or she was sure about his new acquisition and confidently convinces his partner and others. The use of condoms could be mentioned as a new intervention plan. People vary in the speed with which they adopt to a new technique. Those who are eager to adopt are termed innovators or early adopters, while those who are slow are considered unprofessional. The HIV interventions, in this theory were used in the services of respected members of the society, and by trusted and interested population reform members to inform others about adopting a new behavior (Gao et al., 1999).

Combinations of Behavior Therapies

Different combinations of the various behavioral theories described above have been used in different situations, although the behaviors are not guaranteed to be a successful intervention. Other factors also contribute to the success or failure. Successful interventions do not comprise of just delivering facts through a lecture. The interventions are delivered in a precise structure; a few components at a time, until all the planned interventions are received by the staff. Staff and key support personnel must be well trained. The beneficiaries are permitted sufficient opportunities to discuss freely and provide their suggestions about the interventions. The interventions were monitored and evaluated, so that the staff does not get off task, when delivering the HIV prevention measures and protocol (Gao et al., 1999). Interventions were reflective of genuine problems and were culturally appropriate.

Challenges of African American Women

HIV and AIDS have affected the African American race the hardest in the United States (HIV/AIDS Factsheet, 2005). African Americans accounted for 49 percent of the disease, when the specific population was just 13 percent in the U.S. While the proportion of incidence in Dallas was reported as 43 percent or 561, HIV and AIDS cases out of a total number of infected AIDS cases, and (1313) from the HIV/AIDS Surveillance Reports of Dallas County in 2007 (HIV/AIDS Factsheet, 2005). The African American population is 20.26 percent in Dallas, Texas (HIV/AIDS Factsheet, 2005).

The reasons do not simply apply to this ethnic group, but more information applies to the barriers faced by the group (CDC, 2004). Poverty is one main barrier. Unemployment, lack of housing, and the inability to access healthcare and/or treatment may be the other factors associated with poverty. Daily living may be more important than taking care of one's health. This group spends their time and energy to secure food, shelter, and transportation. There is hardly any time for acquiring information about HIV/AIDS, or even any access prevention and/or treatment. Awareness about a new infection was realized as a concern. The belief that it is all an issue of homosexuality may still be the dictum behind the awareness. This group of African American women tends to avoid discussion about the HIV/AIDS disease (CDC, 2004). The disease and the increased prevalence tend to have a negative connotation; therefore, some people tend to remain silent about the HIV/AIDS disease. Behaviors, which promote rash sexual excursions with different partners, increase the prevalence of sexually transmitted diseases. This behavior was related to the larger numbers of females in the population when compared to the male numbers that are reported as 54 percent African American women to 46 percent African American men (CDC, 2004). The number of married females constituted 29 percent, while the married men made up 39 percent of the population (HIV/AIDS Factsheet, 2005). This may be another major causative factor for the high rate of different partners. The households without males could be a reason for women taking the burden of operating single-family homes, and thereby not being able to make ends meet (CDC, 2004). The educational level and lack of access to adequate healthcare and/or medical treatment was indicated as a consequence of poverty and subsequent diverse problems. The negative attitudes, beliefs, and actions against HIV patients were also important in this ethnic group (CDC, 2004).

AIDS has become a disease that affects the African American population and especially the women (AIDS Surveillance Report, 2007). The epidemic has become the biggest killer of the African American community and has been described as the silent killer by many (AIDS Surveillance Report, 2007). All women stand the chance of getting HIV and AIDS. The lack of awareness about the disease coupled with the lack of dialogue among the community members has left this vulnerable population aghast at the outcome.

They are facing an epidemic of important magnitude. All women need to know about the human immunodeficiency (IH-myoo-noh-dif-FISH-uhn-see) virus, or HIV (AIDS Surveillance Report, 2007). HIV causes acquired immunodeficiency syndrome, or AIDS; a disease that weakens the body's ability to fight infection and certain cancers. Having unprotected intercourse is the main way to contract HIV. HIV could be contracted through injection drug use or from mother to baby during pregnancy, childbirth, or breastfeeding (AIDS Surveillance Report, 2007).

Black Homophobia

Operario (2008) reported that AIDS has been attributed to black homophobia. Gay men are not professing their sexuality within the community, while the church marries women for the sake of the putting a family together, despite the black homophobic behavior. These men are described as on the "down low" (Operario, 2008). These men are identified in society as heterosexual men and they deny any homosexual behaviors to their female partners. Prone to feelings of guilt and shame about their sexual behaviors, the men in this particular group hide the fact that they can infect their partners with HIV or other sexually transmitted diseases. In the present context, identifying themselves as a sexual minority of homosexuals might stigmatize them and the families for the rest of their lives.

Black Homophobia is illustrated as a current trend, in which the fear of a loss of black typical identity. This identity is considered as hetero-normative (Kornegay, 2004). Black Homophobia with the concepts of "racism" and "homophobia" have helped identify important social and individual factors that influence the success of prevention activities (Kornegay, 2004).

Kornegay (2004) noted that debauched oppression is evident in black churches according to many heterosexuals who support the view. Kornegay (2004) has reported that the blacks' still suffer from "the unspoken effects of oppression in the form of sex, gender, and race upon the black community and the black church." He believes in the gay theory in helping him challenge the black theology. The perplexing theory was defined as "critical theory concerned principally with cultural deployments of power through social constructions of sexuality and gender" (Kornegay, 2004).

Kelly Brown Douglas attributes black homophobia to black oppression (Kornegay, 2004). Various black thinkers consider homosexuality as a defect in the development of black masculinity and a perversion to manhood (Kornegay, 2004). The lesbian threat is considered as a direct threat to the community's concept of strength, independence, and dominance. The supposition was perceived as a threat to male patriarchy strengthening the "accursed nature of black femininity and homosexuality" (Kornegay, 2004). Kelly Brown says that the white culture has created an image of blacks as sexually unusual people. Kelly encourages the blacks to have more conversation of dialogue about their sexuality and convince others to realize the devastation of HIV/AIDS (Kornegay, 2004). Liberation is encouraged and transformation of awareness may take in sexual discourse and the acceptance of homosexuality must be a consequence.

Effective Interventions for the "Down Low" Men

Malebranche and Wheeler (2005) stated that this effective intervention is not an easy plan for men on the "down low." The men's sexual behaviors, the need for secrecy and confidentiality have elicited concerns from African American women. The emotions of the male and female partners, the possibility of the children's psychological turbulence and the risk of infection are considered as critical and mentioned as possible interventions, for men on the down low (Malebranche & Wheeler, 2005). The intervention is a wise step in saving and preventing HIV/AIDS with this particular group, so that AIDS is not transmitted into the next generation of African American women (Malebranche & Wheeler, 2005).

Just a Behavior-Nothing Serious

Operario (2008) reported that men who engage in relationships with other men believe the preference is a behavior rather than an identity. The behavior makes the men want to hide the nasty tendency from a community, which does not accept the behavior patterns

(Operario, 2008). The term same-sex behavior was considered a behavioral act, as the men secretly hid the behavior and appeared to be straight, heterosexual men in the society. These men believed they are able to have frivolous sex, at any time without a chance of being identified or named "gay," which maybe an insult to their masculinity. The masculine men claim to have no emotional attachment to the male partners, to avoid confrontation in getting into psychological tension and confusion, which may damage the identity of a real-male figure in the community. Operario (2008) posits that these men are not able to hide this twisted behavior, because men do have emotional attachment with other men (Operario, 2008).

The Image of the Breadwinner

A responsible male member is one who was expected to be a breadwinner and provide for his or her families in the community. He or she was not regarded as a responsible person if he loses his heterosexual identity. Another view says that an African American man has forces of oppression and discrimination working against him in America (Operario, 2008). This makes it necessary for a black man to be three times as tough, resilient, and responsible to ward off the malafide forces (Operario, 2008). The pressures of not being able to find a good paying job are also contributors within the community, and therefore the men have to project a tough image. Tradition warrants the picture of a family man, and African American males try to fit into the picture while keeping same-sex behaviors on the sly. There are personal matters, which may affect family members. The matter are kept secret, at least the psychological side, so that others are able to function normally without knowing that the person responsible for making decisions are engaging in risky and intimate behavior (Operario, 2008).

Spontaneous Masculinity Episodes

Operario (2008) posits that there are sudden opportunities, which are presented to males: mixed nightclubs, on the streets, and family gatherings, which may have a chance for anonymous or spontaneous sex episodes. These episodes may occur when they are caught by surprise. These do not have any emotional impact, being just a chance encounter. Maybe a feeling of isolation or depression may have triggered off the encounter (Operario, 2008). Another factor may be the need for closeness and affection, which the men say they do not get from the female partner. Drugs and alcohol may also contribute to an unexpected encounter with other males. Substance abuse may add to the episode and lead one to a behavior, which one normally does not feel comfortable (Operario, 2008). Erotic adventure is another factor, which could lead one to taking risks. A feeling of sexual abandon from the female may make one indulge in uninhibited sex without the use of condoms (Operario, 2008).

The Role of Interventions

Operario (2008) noted that an intervention plan was closely related to the factors that may lead to gay abandon. The first step would involve removing the stigmas attached to homosexual activity (Operario, 2008). This transformation of the behavior of a whole community and the black church is not an easy proposition, but may take place over time. The ability to engage the men, who are considered "at risk" through establishing trust and facilitating open dialogue, may help in the implementation of prevention programs (Operario, 2008). This could be achieved by influencing the church and using peers to reach these people. Getting the men to acknowledge their behaviors, and being able to share the information with their family is another good step but potentially harmful in the context. Consistent use of condoms may work to reduce risks of transmitting HIV. Motivational strategies work better for changing behaviors (Operario, 2008).

Challenges of Women

Women's health and women's rights are subjects for discussion in many communities. There are many challenges for women in regards to the lack of awareness of their rights as women and sexual partners. As reported in Table 1, some of the challenges have been seen as myths people tend to believe about the disease. The HIV/AIDS diseases prevention programs allow women protection from such diseases. The women can learn from the programs, where they are able to negotiate the male partner into using protection. They can use the female condom and explore the right to have safe sex along with pleasure. These are some of the challenges faced by women.

Table 1
Myths/Descriptions about HIV/AIDS

Myth No.	Myth/ Description about HIV/AIDS
1	HIV/AIDS is mostly a disease of homosexual men
2	HIV/AIDS is mostly an African problem
3	HIV/AIDS spreads mostly because of poor moral choices
4	Plenty of money is being spent on fighting HIV/AIDS
5	HIV/AIDS is no longer a problem in the United States
6	Antiretrovirals (ARVs) are widely available
7	A cure exists for HIV/AIDS
8	There is no hope for those with HIV/AIDS
9	If I am not HIV+, the disease does not affect me
10	There is nothing I can do

Note. Adapted from *The Christian Post.* Retrieved from http://christianpost.com/20061130/23769.html.

Feminine Rights

Factors which surround women's problems in AIDS are highlighted in literature. Global and national structural factors that limit the availability of the female condom, use of female oriented prevention technologies and the selection of male partners are considered among the barriers (Mantell, 2008). Frequent harping on the topic might alter the misconceptions, biases, and prejudices of international leaders. Women must also be supported to negotiate for their rights in the world and with their partners. Women must be taught to be discrete and not be deceived on occasion. Their approach should endeavor to include males as active participants (Mantell, 2008).

Female Initiated Methods

Women tend to be uninformed of the outcomes of the need to protect themselves against AIDS (Mantell, 2008). Physical and chemical barriers are to reduce to the chance of HIV/AIDS. Microbicides and cervical barriers are tested for efficacy. The female condom was established as an efficient method of preventing pregnancy and sexually transmitted diseases (Hoffman, Mantell, Exner & Stein, 2004). The AIDS pandemic is not just a matter of transmission, infection, or therapy, but involves the family. The pandemic is a universal risk for women of all races (UNAIDS, 2005).

The Acceptance of the Female Condom

Some countries promote abstinence and faithfulness for the purpose of HIV/AIDS prevention (Mantell, Stein, & Susser, 2008). Any condom use, least of all the female condom, was not accepted in such a situation. Free availability of the female condoms in pharmacies, clinics, supermarkets, restrooms, vending machines and through social marketing would help in reaching all women who need them (Mantell, 2008). A large amount of funds needs to be resourced for this measure to be successful. International conferences and policy makers hardly look upon the condom as a possible solution (Mulama, 2007). Government apathy, inaction, and lack of a coherent plan to boost the female condom as an effective means of reducing HIV infection are obvious (Mulama, 2007). The possible prevention solution has made the female condom inaccessible and used scarcely (Mulama, 2007). Another structural barrier was the lower cost of the male condom, which is 20 times less costly. The potential of reducing the number of AIDS case was increased with the usage of female condom to ensure protection of the female and offspring too. The cost of projected cases should be sufficient to consider the usefulness of the female condom (Cravero, 2006). The number of averted cases should be another reason favoring the female condom (Dowdy, Sweat, & Holtgrave, 2006). Botswana, Zimbabwe, Ghana, and Zambia promote the female condom because of the potential good results (Mantell, 2008). A strange factor noticed was that sponsors have funded research of microbicides and vaccines while ignoring the female condom (Mantell, 2008). Others have funded the HIV prevention technologies of male circumcision, herpes HSV-2 suppression, cervical barriers, and vaccines (Mantell, 2008). Cost and aesthetic judgment are blamed, as the causes for non-acceptance of the female condom for policy makers rather than women at risk (Mantell, 2008). Further, government and community support, sufficient funds, incorporating the female barrier methods into public service venues address family planning, drug therapy, tuberculosis, hepatitis, HIV prevention, and care and treatment programs, are enabling environments for marketing the female condoms (Mantell, 2008).

Control and Leadership Knowledge of Women

Women using female initiated techniques are more self-reliable and autonomous (Telles, Diaz, Souto & Page-Schafer, 2006). As Telles, et al. (2006) stated, they are in a position to improve their dialogue and negotiate with their male partners. There is increasing consciousness of women's rights (Mantell, 2008). The empowerment of women through knowledge, awareness, and ability to utilize the resources available are the leadership qualities that must be employed in order to become effective against HIV/AIDS prevention.

Discretion in Female Initiated Methods

Some men see the method of female initiated techniques as a license for women to be promiscuous (Mantell et al., 2008). The reality is that the female condom empowers the women to decide how to accommodate their partners and yet protect themselves sexually (Mantell, 2008). There are some countries that insist on a 100 percent use of the male condom especially among intimate relationships (Mantell, 2008).

Some women prefer the diaphragm and microbicides rather than the female condom as they can be used discretely (Terris-Prestholt et al., 2006). Mantell (2008) reports the majority of new HIV infections are contracted from husbands who have extra-marital affairs or many partners. The discrete use of preventative methods ensures lasting or secure marital relationships (Mantell, 2008).

The Male Partners' Acceptance

Men face a difficulty in accepting a female initiated preventive method. Partner influence is a key factor in the new initiated use (Mantell, 2008). Some men are happy that the female takes responsibility in using the condom. Sometimes the female condom comes in useful when the male refuses to use a male one. The time is more evident that the male partner should support the female initiated method or the female's usage of the female condom. Some men prefer the diaphragm, because the preventive instrument did not feel like the female condom or male condom during the act. Women have commented that the condom reduces their pleasure physically, but the feeling of relief from getting pregnant was enhanced (Mantell, 2008). Several American women claim more pleasure for both partners with the female condom. With the AIDS threat, the need to incorporate safer sex into pleasure along with the prevention of pregnancy or disease is important (Higgins & Hirsch, 2007). As women's HIV protection depends on the male partner's cooperation, there are barriers of acceptance with different methods. These methods empower women and at the same time are accepted by the male, and may be used for best results. In order to promote the usage of the female condom, both parties should explore further ideals regarding the outcomes (Mantell, 2008).

Gender Bias

Gender bias must be intercepted at the global, government and media levels. Women must be central to all decisions involving the prevention of HIV/AIDS. Prejudices about female barrier methods should be removed in developed and resource limited nations (Mantell, 2008). Women should be supported to select their barrier method from many options. Women must first be informed about their rights and the available methods. Men should be targeted and informed about current preventive information. The phases promote the use of female initiated methods, so that men are aware of the preventive measures.

Current Literature

Hoy-Ellis (2007) reports AIDS as a terminal (incurable) disease many years ago. Today, AIDS has been reported as a chronic (constant) but manageable disease (Hoy-Ellis, 2007). A study mentions the perceptions of patients are divided: 41 percent considered AIDS as chronic and 37 percent as terminal (Hoy-Ellis, 2007). A decision could not be made for 17 percent, of the patients. The results showed that the more educated person could see AIDS as chronic. Those who felt discrimination due to ethnicity spoke of AIDS as a terminal disease (Hoy-Ellis, 2007). There are about 58 percent of the people living with AIDS and who had medications considered the disease as chronic while 29 percent perceived AIDS as terminal and 11 percent were not sure. Among the informal support partners who had medications, 55 percent claimed the disease to be chronic, while 28 percent thought AIDS was terminal.

As Hoy-Ellis (2007) reported some patients commented, "If they did not die of AIDS, they would probably die of the medications and thereby still consider the disease terminal." The medicines do not improve the health of those with HIV, which is considered terminal. Based on some of the people, the disease was chronic or terminal based on knowledge, awareness, and personal experiences (Hoy-Ellis, 2007). There were 54 percent of persons living with AIDS personally thought that it is chronic while 40 percent termed AIDS as terminal. There are 62 percent of the informal support group who cited personal experience, also considered AIDS chronic, and the remainder of the support group considered AIDS as terminal. Many people living with it and in the informal support group who wished for a cure believed it was chronic. Education, on the disease is influenced by the people generally to believe in the chronic view. HIV/AIDS can be described as a disease of ambiguity and change (Hoy-Ellis, 2007).

The awareness of the HIV/AIDS changes over the years as innovations in treatment are developed. The changing trend about the disease, the need to openly discuss treatment, availability of medicines (free for most people who cannot afford the medicines), and adhering to medications faithfully could influence the outcome of the disease. Healthcare professionals should be trained on the latest knowledge about the HIV/AIDS disease, which could help disseminate information directly to the patients (Hoy-Ellis, 2007).

Changes in Methods of Assessing Epidemiology

Methodological changes include the attempt to understand the epidemiology of HIV/AIDS. Doing more population based questionnaires, extending sentinel surveillance to include more sites in more countries, adjusting the mathematic models used are the main changes brought about in 2007 (WHO, 2007). There are about 6,800 persons who are believed to become infected, and 5,700 die daily because of improper access to prevention and treatment. Obviously, this disease is a major health problem. People are living longer with the HIV/AIDS disease, which has increased the number of people who are living with HIV infection. A small reduction in deaths has been noticed in some countries. The reduction in the mortality of HIV cases is due to the improved anti-retroviral treatment techniques and better access (WHO, 2007). These drugs delay the progression of AIDS, as the disease changes into a chronic condition (Guthrie, 2005). The better quality of life and the delay in the end stages of the disease contribute to this reduction. Two patterns of epidemics are seen. The Sub Saharan Africa is the most seriously affected and exhibits a generalized epidemic while the rest of the world shows the epidemics to involve high-risk individuals in high-risk populations like homosexual men, injection drug users, sex workers and their partners (WHO, 2007). The trends of incidence are showing a decline in many countries where prevention techniques are fruitful, even in some parts of Sub Saharan Africa (WHO, 2007).

North America had an incidence of 1.3 million where 46,000 were the new cases. Deaths had been 21,000 in 2007 (WHO, 2007). The figures are similar to those of the previous years. The number of men and women living with HIV was 15.4 million each. The ratio of men to women was the same as in 2001. The proportions of women to men in many countries varied. The Sub Saharan Africa had 61 percent women while in the Caribbean (43 percent), Central Asia (26 percent), Eastern Europe (26 percent) and Asia (29 percent), the proportion of women was less (WHO, 2007).

New Data and Packages

The Estimation and Projection Package (EPP), WORKBOOK, and Spectrum are the new instruments for estimating incidence. The generation of an HIV prevalence curve, listed with the age specific demographics illustrates mortality. Sentinel surveillance, questionnaires, and special studies have provided improved data. Many new assumptions added into the software tools were used in reporting the incidences. The HIV Surveillance systems in some countries are insufficient and produce gaps (WHO, 2007).

HIV incidence can be understood by watching the trends in 18- to 24-year-old pregnant women who would have recently acquired the infection. Women pose being influenced less by anti-retroviral treatments and mortality like the older women. Recent information shows a decrease of incidence in 11 out of 15 of the most affected countries studied.

Recent Interventions

Advancing HIV Prevention (AHP)

The Center for Disease Control and Prevention started the Advancing HIV Prevention (AHP) in 2003 (CDC Factsheet, 2008). The CDC has imposed four strategies, which involve AHP. The HIV testing has been a routine procedure in medical care. Diagnosing HIV outside medical settings is possible, but may not be accurate as the regulations of the government. Preventive methods for infected persons have been made possible. Perinatal HIV transmission has been decreased (CDC Factsheet, 2008).

African American Workgroup

The CDC is initiating the African American HIV/AIDS work group (CDC Factsheet, 2008). The objective is to have prevention and intervention activities that are directed towards African American women. Community leaders are working with this ethnic group in order to motivate about awareness and help decrease the incidence of HIV/AIDS in the group.

Rapid Testing and Evaluation in Colleges

The CDC institutes rapid HIV testing and evaluation. Testing and evaluation is implemented in colleges historically having mostly African Americans. New projects are in force, for improving the HIV testing among African American women. Studies are being conducted by the Brothers Y. Hermanos that help to identify risk promoting and risk reducing sexual behaviors in Los Angeles, New York and Philadelphia. Such studies are being conducted in Texas too. African American women studies have examined relationship dynamics and the cultural, psychosocial, and behavioral factors associated with HIV infection' (CDC HIV/AIDS Factsheet, 2008).

Minority AIDS Initiative

Information was disseminated through Minority AIDS initiative. Sufficient funds are mobilized for the preventive policies to help community-based organizations provide services. Telephone help lines, internet resources, and programs in barbershops are available in order to reduce risks, with social support to help disadvantaged African American men and women (CDC Factsheet, 2008). Social marketing campaigns that focus on HIV testing, perinatal transmission and the reduction of transmission to partners are rampant. Interventions are being disseminated to those in need of information and/or treatment.

Sisters Informing Sisters about Topics on AIDS—SISTA

Sisters informing sisters about topics on AIDS (SISTA) are prevention programs with peer facilitators that help African American women, who are at risk gain social skills training. Many Men Many Voices (3MV) is another prevention program that helps homosexual men reduce their risks of being infected. Popular Opinion Leader (POL) is another program that identifies and trains leaders in the community to spread messages in the African American population (CDC Factsheet, 2008). These organizations represent healthy relationships, represented by groups that serve women that are infected with HIV/AIDS.

Women Involved in Life Learning from Other Women—WILLOW

Women Involved in Life Learning from other women (WILLOW) has skills training interventions for infected women. The HIV/AIDS training increases the awareness of risky behaviors, teaches negotiation for safer sex and condom use. The program provides information about shelters for HIV/AIDS women (CDC Factsheet, 2008). CDC provides training for researchers from minority groups, such as African American women.

MARI—Minority HIV/AIDS Research Initiative

The Minority HIV/AIDS Research Initiative (MARI) encourages partnerships between epidemiologists and researchers of the minority races, and those who work between the African American and other minority groups (Centers for Disease Control and Prevention, 2008). There is over $2 million spent every year on research and prevention measures in the communities. The goals of the MARI program are: (1) To build HIV prevention research capacity in Black and Hispanic communities in which little research is conducted by partnering with and developing new investigators in these communities to address pertinent research questions; (2) To engage in career development and provide research opportunities; and (3) To develop and conduct HIV epidemiologic prevention research in the form of limited case-controlled, cross-sectional, or qualitative projects that have public health relevance to Black and Hispanic communities (National Prevention Information Network, 2008).

The Multi-Sectorial Approach

Health care dealing with HIV infections in the community benefited from a multisectorial approach (Toro, 2006). A four-pronged objective was planned for situational analysis, research and planning, and implementation and evaluation. Teamwork formed the backbone of such a project. Some advantages are the gaps in services, which were assessed immediately and prevented early. Concrete improvements were ensured with this new approach (Toro, 2006). Similar endeavors are illustrated in many places under different names: partnership approach (Berkowitz, 2004), multi-disciplinary team (Chafe, 2004), community based effort (Casey et al., 2004), and multi-sectorial collaboration. The multi-sectorial approach involves all sectors of society including the government, businesses, social organizations, and people living with AIDS. This response requires the self-confidence to mobilize political backing and leadership qualities to develop, coordinate, and sustain partnerships. New methods of working evolved along the way. Frequently reassessing situations and strengthening all sectors to make the individual contributions effective determined the success of the project (Toro, 2006). Group dynamics involved adjustments among the many strong leaders during interactions so that ample respect for personal and professional identity, recognition, appreciation and limitation of strong personalities were upheld and the interactions became learning experiences (Toro, 2006). The differences in this approach were that all the decisions, objectives, policies, budgets, administrative affairs, research, monitoring, and evaluation had the recommendations from the team. The leaders are facilitators and coordinators during the group dynamics. The strategies caused the team to become motivated and interested in prevention. The team used communications monthly meetings, telephone calls, formal and informal environments for meetings in order to build an active Internet communication system. The difficult situations arose in spite of the arrangements that were along the way. The achievements included the formation and maintenance of the team itself. The unique method of thinking evolved after a few interactions helped in the existence of a fully functional and committed team. The working style was used to revise interventions for success of the program, and this model would be expected to last for five years, as the program progresses.

Opportunistic Infections

Opportunistic infections are the clinical presentations of the HIV/AIDS disease in spite of the highly active antiretroviral therapy (HAART) and these cause mortality. The HAART therapy transformed the lives of many HIV infected people in the 1990s. HIV related morbidity and mortality greatly reduces following the institution of this therapy. Peumocystitis jiroveci still causes a large number of deaths due to pneumonia (Gebo et al., 2005). Opportunistic infections are related to increased risks of progression of disease, mortality and health care costs (Hanna, 2007). Delays in the diagnosis of HIV infection cause rapid onset of opportunistic infections and prevent prophylaxis and HAART being effective (Hanna, 2007).

In a survey conducted in 2000 in New York, the results proved that 27.4 percent of AIDS cases have one opportunistic infection while the remaining 72.6 percent had a reduction of CD4+ lymphocytes to below 200 microl as the AIDS defining event. The incidence of one or more opportunistic infections was found more in African Americans (Hanna, 2007). The highest incidence of opportunistic infections was seen in patients with late diagnosis. Persons who had HAART within the recent 12 months had lesser risk of these infections. Many persons are found to have reached the AIDS stage without having known about their disease for a long time (Hanna et al., p. 268).

The most common opportunistic infections are pnuemocystitis carinii pneumonia, tuberculosis, wasting syndrome, candidiasis, and toxoplasmosis of the brain. The infections accounted for 88 percent of AIDS-defining opportunistic infections in 2000 (Hanna, 2007). The infections may have been prevented with HAART or prophylaxis. There are 80 percent of opportunistic infections that may be prevented with HAART; and uninsured or under-insured people may benefit from the free HAART medicines (Hanna, 2007).

What Works

The decline seen in the prevalence of HIV/AIDS after the year 2000 was attributed to many factors. HIV prevalence must be simultaneously correlated in order to reduce HIV incidence, from a number of new cases to make HIV/AIDS an important finding. Prevalence may be lower, due to stable incidence and increasing mortality (Pankhurst, 2008). The reductions were traced to behavioral changes in the general population. Behavioral changes need not always be responses to national policy changes.

The change would be better suited to reduce HIV/AIDS and help reduce the risk behavior and new infections that cause the lowered prevalence of HIV. HIV prevalence was one component that could explain what works. The decline in this figure is evident and the decline is occurring globally. The timing and extent of the decline has varied with population and area. The picture may not be representative of all the countries in the world (Pankhurst, 2008).

The component parts of new HIV infections are more important (Pankhurst, 2008). When the prevalence decreases, HIV/AIDS becomes important to note whether the disease has occurred due to lesser new infections. HIV/AIDS information may be used to determine, because there are many factors to encourage the changes.

Knowing how behaviors have changed during the prior years has led to the present revelation about HIV/AIDS awareness and considered the third component (Pankhurst, 2008). Behavioral data is difficult to obtain. Questionnaires assess behaviors in different manners with different questions. The answers obtained may vary. A question about the use of condoms may elicit an answer that is different from the original question (Pankhurst, 2008). The second format would probably give a more relevant answer for HIV inquiry (Pankhurst, 2008). The number of lifetime partners may be less relevant than the number of concurrent partners, as these results have not changed for statistics purposes (Pankhurst, 2008).

The fourth component of the causes of behavior changes implies that certain strategies implemented brought about these behavior changes. The diversity of interventions and different applications in different countries makes HIV/AIDS reporting difficult. Sometimes the topics of HIV/AIDS are the social setup and interactions are the behavior changes. Social, economic, cultural and political factors may be working together to change behaviors (Pankhurst, 2008). A specific cause of HIV/AIDS was not identified in this study.

The fifth component of responsible policies did not affect HIV prevalence. This was because interventions for reducing infection rates were usually not influenced by policy changes. There is yet no coordination between the two aspects. Speculation was natural to attribute a reduced prevalence to the latest policy changes (Pankhurst, 2008). Pankhurst's study posits that HIV/AIDS is not easy to understand or attributes a reduction prevalence or incidence of HIV to specific components or what works.

Survival Benefits of AIDS Care

Pankhurst (2008) reports studies of the cumulative survival benefits from health care to AIDS patients. The health care information provided includes opportunistic infection prophylaxis, treatment with ART (Antiretroviral Therapy), and prevention of mother to child transmission (Walensky, 2006). The individual survival increased 0.26 years from the prophylaxis of Pneumocystitis jiroveci pneumonia alone. The effective ART showed differing number of years' survival depicting the variation in effectiveness of the ART instituted. The human being survival increases from 7.81, 11.05, 11.57, and 13.33 years, when compared to the absence of treatment (Walensky, 2006). The treatment for patients with AIDS in the United States shows a survival benefit of 2.8 million years. The prevention of mother to child transmission saves 2,900 children from infections equivalent to 137,000 additional years of survival benefit. Advances in treatment of AIDS saved 3 million lives in the U.S. (Walensky, 2006).

Leadership

Self-leadership was the second focus of this study. Self-leadership has been defined as the process of a person to improve his or her self-motivations and influence his or her self-direction to behave in desirable ways (Konradt, 2008). Several theories relate to self-leadership: the social cognition theory, theories of self-control and self-regulation (Konradt, 2008).

The self-management theory was based on behavioral theories. This leadership theory has been mostly associated with self-leadership. The strategies include behavior focused, natural reward, cognitive ability, and thought pattern strategies (Konradt, 2008). The behavior-focused strategies are believed to increase self-awareness. Positive desirable behaviors were enhanced and negative behavior were restrained (Houghton and Neck, 2002). The leader sets the goals, rewards, makes observations, punishes, and cues

(Konradt, 2008). The natural rewarding activities help to develop competence, self-control, and purpose. Dysfunctional and irrational beliefs were identified through self-leadership (Manz & Neck, 2004). The existing and irrational thoughts have been changed in a self-leadership strategy. Positive relationships have been recognized between thorough self-leadership and more effective leadership and outcomes, when one can identify and change his or her normal patterns of thinking through self-directed leadership (Houghton & Neck, 2006). Individual self-management has a positive effect on team performance (Konradt, 2008).

Self-leadership was described as a motivational theory where self motivation develops an intense and persistent organizational behavior. Behavioral and cognitive strategies would influence this change. The motivation theory was derived from the expectancy-value theory where behavior is actually a function of the required expectations and goals to which one is working (Hertel, Konradt, & Orlikowski, 2004).

Self-leadership techniques increase self-efficacy as people become more confident through self-control. Self-leadership contributes to team performance and positive behaviors that do not cause any discrepancies in teamwork, which should be practiced (Konradt, 2008). A self-leadership strategy affects self-efficacy, which directly affects performance. The characteristics of the team and intra team processes promoted motivation through self-influence and individual performance. When the individual was on task, the team was well defined and performance measures were improved by individual self-leadership. The intra team processes improved with the individual self-leadership behaviors (Konradt, 2008).

Conclusion

The literature illustrated how much information African American women in the Dallas/Fort Worth areas of Texas; know about HIV/AIDS awareness, with the use of self-leadership skills. Tarakeshwar (2008) found that the literature on AIDS was vast. The results are congruent to HIV/AIDS as more data was reported by the Centers for Disease Control and Prevention, and other peer-reviewed sources. AIDS is a subject that reveals several changes in the presence of the disease. Prevention techniques stem from the large-scale ones to innovative techniques that focus on small populations. The populations targeted are the partners of HIV positive men (Tarakeshwar, 2008), incarcerated men (Grinstead, 2008), and African American people (CDC HIV/AIDS Factsheet, 2008), college students, and partners of people who have enrolled in injection drug abuse rehabilitation programs. Female initiated techniques are being stressed as an awareness concept (Mantell, 2008). The African American community has to rid themselves of class oppression and their women of gender oppression, and the concept of black homophobia as a first step towards reducing the incidence among them (Operario, 2008). The incorporation of behavior models, preventive methods with dissemination of information through peers or peer education may help reduce the incidence of HIV/AIDS. More important, members of the African American community, especially their women or even the white community need to know about the progresses and changes that are occurring in the incidence, transmission patterns, medical treatment, prevention techniques and peer education or support groups available for their help in relationship to HIV/AIDS.

Summary

The main idea about awareness of HIV/AIDS has seen progressive changes. The reduction in incidence in recent years has contributed many factors of successful preventive techniques. There are more effective HAART techniques for controlling the opportunistic infections, and ensuring that more people with the disease stay alive (Guthrie, 2005), with the use of different techniques. These techniques have been employed for reducing incidence of HIV/AIDS (WHO, 2007).

Self-leadership was the theoretical method selected for organizing this qualitative study of grounded theory design. After highlighting the literature that embodies the innovative changes associated with HIV/AIDS, this study was justified. The study also revealed awareness issues among African American women participants.

In this chapter, there was a disclosure of literature pertaining to the research questions, the history of HIV/AIDS, behavioral theories for HIV prevention, and the challenges of African American women in Dallas and Fort Worth, Texas. A historical overview with current findings and a discussion of gaps in the literature was also included. Chapter 3 revealed the research and instrument design, and data analysis of this study.

CHAPTER 3

RESEARCH METHOD

The purpose of this qualitative grounded theory study was to explore the lack of HIV/AIDS awareness in African American women in the Dallas and Fort Worth areas of Texas. Quantification was not possible in the present situation where the intention was to elicit new subjective information from the participants. The research design was discovery-oriented and holistic (Forman et al., 2008). The appropriateness of the methodology and design was qualitative, which means that reasoning about appropriateness involves the use of assumptions. The assumptions (questionnaires) are the controls used to reason about the validity or appropriateness of using the individual questions. The assumptions were used to express the relevance of awareness about HIV/AIDS. Reasonable constraints between illustrating assumptions comprise an important section of introducing the theoretical framework.

An example of revealing assumptions was to assume that most African American women were not aware of the effects of the disease, because so many of them are dying from the disease. In other words, when a qualitative questionnaire was distributed, there was equal distribution of knowledge, because everyone received the same information. Having prior knowledge about HIV/AIDS allowed the participants an opportunity to complete more questions. This study revealed information about the depth of the lack of awareness of HIV/AIDS. A goal of eliciting the lack of awareness regarding HIV/AIDS through a discovery oriented and holistic approach was achieved through a qualitative and interpretative research and a grounded theory design. The design was completed with the use of questionnaires that were devised for the purpose of assessing self-leadership qualities. A sample of 30 African American women was selected for this study. Their ages were between 18 and 54 and the women had a minimum of a high school education. The ability to read and write English was also a criterion. The questionnaires elicited information about why this community of African American women was not responding favorably to the worldwide campaign of HIV/AIDS awareness. This group did not respond to HIV/AIDS awareness, as other groups in the communities. The questionnaires showed explicit information. Unfortunately, the participants did not ask detail questions about the disease. Harris and Holdt (1997) believed that African American women were the scapegoats of class oppression and/or racial discrimination or gender oppression in the Texas areas. This qualitative study indicated some new information regarding the lack of awareness through the inclusion of questions requiring open-ended answers that encouraged African American women through concerted awareness about the HIV/AIDS disease.

Research Method Appropriateness

The qualitative research method revealed in depth information, which explored the awareness of HIV/AIDS, among African American women. The aim of the research was to reveal awareness from the participants concerning how the HIV/AIDS disease affects the lives of women. The information gathering was open-ended qualitative research. The behaviors and social practices of African American women were investigated. The holistic and discovery-oriented approach required a qualitative technique rather than a quantitative. Questionnaires were open-ended and provided more detail from variable responses (Patton, 2002). Open-ended questions had the advantage of eliciting answers from the participants that would convey the women's perceptions of HIV/AIDS. There were no pre-determined viewpoints that could be impinged upon the participants. The answers from each participant varied in qualitative research as the information revealed an idea about awareness. The explicit nature of the answers added value to the study. The participants divulged information, which maybe quoted in future research studies. The participant's depth of emotion was conveyed. This study revealed a better understanding of how African American women's environments were organized through experiences, thoughts, perceptions, and the extent of awareness with regard to the subject of HIV/AIDS. Qualitative research provided the framework required for this current study. Each participant provided different answers, while a wealth of knowledge was gained from the study.

Questionnaires were the simplest form of data collection; and the information provided the opportunity to explore the results. Questions were user-friendly, so that the participants were relaxed and at ease, while divulging, such critical information. The topic about HIV/AIDS added to the capacity, for a wealth of information to make appropriate conclusions. Details about African American women's attitudes and behaviors in relationship were obtained through a questionnaire. Awareness levels in the community served to reveal different behaviors, which was a concern for African American women. The opinions and attitudes, about how the women were affected by vigorous campaigns affected responses. Whether the women felt the stigma of class oppression and gender oppression are revelations that were believed to evolve from this study. The information was of an emergent design and revealed awareness about HIV/AIDS (Harris & Holdt, 1997).

The responses from the participants revealed a disadvantage, which was reflected on the questionnaire and added depth to this study. The research method allowed the participants an opportunity to reveal information without observer dependency. This current study was based on participants who had a high school education; and understood the importance of giving true answers. The questionnaires were simple, requiring only a yes or *no* answer or crossing-out of the wrong statements. Only a few questions required open-ended answers. Open-ended questions were predetermined with the object of refraining from putting the participants through stress about cooperating with the research. The participation in answering the questions added to African American women's level of information on the topic about HIV/AIDS awareness. The answers to the question set four (4), included the open-ended questions that helped the women think critically about intimate relationships. For example, a participant inquired about free treatment or where to get the treatment based on the answers to the user-friendly open-ended questions.

Qualitative research methods were used to gather and illustrate the results. This study does not focus on quantitative research. Specifically, in experimental quantitative research, the subjects were measured before and after a treatment. Treatment and/or any intervention were not involved in this present study. The experimental quantitative research was not applicable (Creswell, 2002). Future study could be done using the experimental quantitative method for research using the basic ideas obtained from this qualitative study, followed by interventions to increase awareness and then reassessing the awareness. A control group without interventions could also be instituted and studied. The mixed variety of research employs a quantitative and qualitative research. A mixed variety was not required as the objective of this study were to elicit maximum unknown information from a selected sample of 30 African American women in the Dallas and Fort Worth areas of Texas.

Research Design Appropriateness

The grounded theory design was selected for this study. This design originated from Glaser and Strauss's theory of constant comparison. Glaser and Strauss (1967) defines a theory as a set of well-developed categories, which are consistent through statements of relationship to form a theoretical framework to explain some relevant social, psychological, educational, nursing or other phenomenon. This design does not begin with a theory. The theory evolved during this study process because of continuous data collection and analysis (Coleman & O'Connor, 2007). The belief was that the evolved theory was likely to resemble reality, rather than a theory formed out of experience and speculation at the start of a research as in a quantitative research.

Several steps were incorporated to ensure the evolution of a practical theory. Coding strategies were incorporated into the analytical process. The information obtained from the questionnaires was critiqued into concepts, or units of meaning. The data were rearranged and reevaluated for design appropriateness. There appeared a core category and a variable, which were seen frequently, throughout this study. This analysis guided the study into an emergent theory.

The Question of Ethics

Interaction Institute for Social Change (2009) reported that evidence about the study revealed private information from the participants. Necessary precautions were in place to convince the participants about the genuineness of the study, and the future implications (Interaction Institute for Social Change, 2009). Then, the participants were issued an informed consent letter of authorization that allowed them to participate and reveal intimate, private, and confidential information.

Demographic Data

Demographic data were collected at the second visit and letters of consent for participating in the research were distributed. As reported by the Interaction Institute for Social Change (2010), the demographic questionnaire revealed information about the participant's gender, age, highest educational level, race/ethnicity, which allowed them to self-identify themselves about the awareness of HIV/AIDS in the African American community. The example of the demographic questionnaire has been exhibited as Appendix A and Appendix B. All participants were African American women from Dallas and Fort Worth areas of Texas as listed in Table 2.

Table 2
Demographic/Geographic and Ethnicity Result

Participant	Gender	Age	Education	Geographic Location	Ethnicity
P1	Female	52	Degree	Dallas County	African American
P2	Female	22	Current College Student	Dallas County	African American

P3	Female	27	Current College Student	Dallas County	African American
P4	Female	25	Current College Student	Dallas County	African American
P5	Female	21	Current College Student	Dallas County	African American
P6	Female	21	Current College Student	Dallas County	African American
P7	Female	41	Degree & Current College Student	Dallas County	African American
P8	Female	20	Current College Student	Dallas County	African American
P9	Female	21	Current College Student	Dallas County	African American
P10	Female	23	Current College Student	Dallas County	African American
P11	Female	25	Current College Student	Dallas County	African American
P12	Female	24	Current College Student	Dallas County	African American
P13	Female	20	Current College Student	Dallas County	African American
P14	Female	22	Current College Student	Dallas County	African American
P15	Female	21	Current College Student	Dallas County	African American
P16	Female	20	Current College Student	Tarrant County	African American
P17	Female	23	Current College Student	Tarrant County	African American
P18	Female	21	Current College Student	Tarrant County	African American
P19	Female	20	Current College Student	Tarrant County	African American
P20	Female	25	Current College Student	Tarrant County	African American
P21	Female	38	Current College Student	Tarrant County	African American

P22	Female	22	Current College Student	Tarrant County	African American
P23	Female	27	Current College Student	Tarrant County	African American
P24	Female	23	Current College Student	Tarrant County	African American
P25	Female	32	Degree & Current College Student	Tarrant County	African American
P26	Female	21	Current College Student	Tarrant County	African American
P27	Female	20	Current College Student	Tarrant County	African American
P28	Female	24	Current College Student	Tarrant County	African American
P29	Female	21	Current College Student	Tarrant County	African American
P30	Female	20	Current College Student	Tarrant County	African American

Population

A simple questionnaire was implemented to obtain a representative sample of the target population in order to recruit persons that directly reflected the population. The selected population was African American women from the Dallas and Fort Worth areas of Texas. To ensure that African American women were questioned, only African American students who attended Dallas and Tarrant counties colleges were part of a targeted sample, as shown in Table 2.

Sampling Method

The evidence from the study focused on African American women in Dallas and Fort Worth areas because of the rate of African Americans women dying of HIV/AIDS. This study addressed an increase of the deadly pandemic of HIV/AIDS in the Dallas/Fort Worth areas. The HIV/AIDS pandemic has been proved as one of the devastating social conditions in these cities (Johnson, 2007).

The sample for this study consisted of African American women, 18-54 years of age, who resided in the Dallas and Fort Worth areas of Texas. According to Tuan (2006), from 2000 through 2003, HIV and AIDS rates for African American women were 19 times the rates for white women (Tuan, 2006). African American women accounted for 67 percent of all new AIDS cases among women in 2003, while white females accounted for 15 percent (Tuan, 2006). African American women constituted 13 percent of the U.S. female population and whites constituted at least 66 percent (Census Bureau, 2004). To ensure that a small sample of African American women are questioned; community colleges in both cities were part of a targeted sample. A convenience sample consisted of participants from the following community colleges:

1. Eastfield Community College/Dallas County.
2. Tarrant County College/Fort Worth, Texas.

Sampling

The sample for this current study consisted of 30 African American women who were members of participating community colleges, and appear to be African American/Black women. Data were collected via self-administered questionnaires, which were completed at the participating colleges. Data were analyzed using descriptive information to gather the results of the level of HIV/AIDS awareness from African American women suggested by a theoretical model. The research presented the communities with critical insight into behavioral and/or social trends of African American women's motivation for, and involvement in HIV/AIDS related awareness, which may lead to the development of targeted community-based HIV/AIDS awareness programs.

For this procedure, a random selection of African American women was selected. This method involved the selection of the sample at random from the sampling population through the use of questionnaires (Saunders, Lewis & Thornhill, 2003). Questionnaires were given to each participant. Confidential envelopes were given to African American women, who were in the selected population, until the sample size was reached.

The time constraints and compromises were often necessary in the sample frame. In such cases, it was important to realize the limitations that resulted from a sample selection procedure. The proposed sample utilized African American women were from Dallas and Fort Worth Texas.

Geographic Location

This dissertation integrates geographic information mitigating awareness about HIV/AIDS from African American women. The awareness issues have been narrowed to, two specific geographical locations (Dallas and Fort Worth, Texas) in hope to gain the desired results. The locations were selected because of an increase in deaths with African American women, which have ranked high in these areas (see Figure 3).

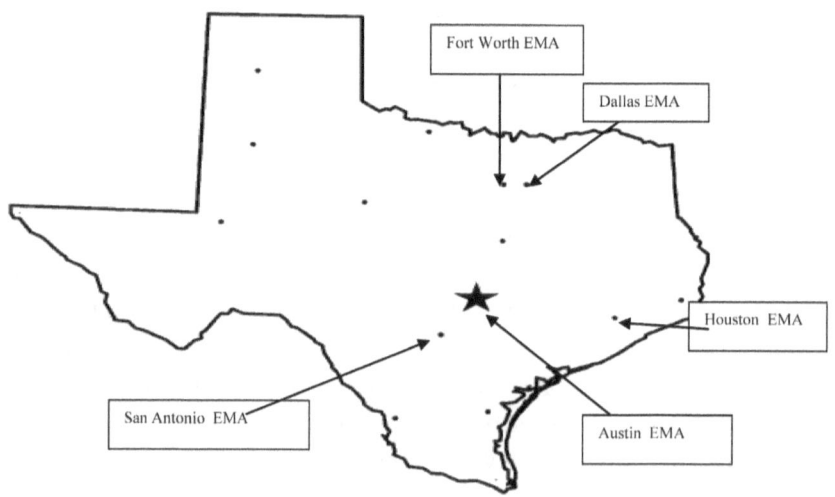

Figure 3. Geographic Areas of Interest/Texas, 2007. Adapted from "HIV/AIDS in Texas," 2007, 2009, *Texas Integrated Epidemiologic Profile for HIV/AIDS Prevention and Services Planning,* p. 14. Retrieved from http://www.dshs.state.tx.us/hivstd/planning/EpiProfile.pdf

The analysis and results were taken from Dallas and Fort Worth, Texas, as the demographic location for this research. These locations formed the platform for gathering the data. The demographic locations served as the basis for creating awareness and allowing the information to penetrate the community, because the sampling areas were known for one of the highest estimated rates of African American women living with HIV/AIDS (CDC, 2004). Data were gathered from these cities; and, therefore, was not generalized. Evidence from the participant's was limited to those persons who were present at the scheduled time(s) of the questionnaire instrument. Only women from the two cities were allowed to participate. The participants were African American women registered as college students at Dallas and/or Tarrant county community colleges. They were between the ages of 18-54, which allowed them to participate in this current study.

Data Collection

This current study was conducted in Dallas and Fort Worth, Texas. Data collection consisted of semi-structured interviews, which were used to ensure integrity of this study (Goldsmith, 2005). Primary data were collected by administering individual, in-depth, semi-structured interviews to explore knowledge levels from African American women in regards to self-awareness about HIV/AIDS. The study participants were asked to reveal intimate, confidential, and personal information about HIV/AIDS awareness. The sampling frame for individuals comprised those women attending college, African American, and between the ages of 18-54 years of age.

Although, the study results could not predict the exact sample size, the study results provided successful information from gathering 15 women per city. Analyses were conducted interactively with data collection to inform the purposeful sampling strategy. Specifically, the informed consent process was not a single event or a form to sign. Rather, the process was an interactive educational process that took place, between the investigator and the subject (Collaborative Institutional Training Initiative, 2005).

Analysis steps followed traditional grounded theory approaches. The results were compared with traditional knowledge about awareness theory. The results were used to inform the participants about different programs on HIV/AIDS awareness. The developing theory was developed to inform women about access to prevention theory, in order to better design empirical research on awareness (McMillan, 1996). The research was an important tool to help community leaders design programs that may help facilitate African American women's needs with respect to awareness about HIV/AIDS.

More women have become infected with HIV since the disease was first reported in the early 1980s (McMillan, 1996). Today one in four Americans living with HIV/AIDS are women. African American women are the most affected. HIV/AIDS is the leading cause of death for African American women aged 25 to 34 (McMillan, 1996).

Informed Consent

Students from Dallas and Tarrant county community colleges were evaluated in this study. The department leaders were contacted, and informed about the nature of the study. The directors were informed about the risks, (beneficence, no harm), with this research study, and the results from this study are not targeted as research to be shared with outside affiliates. The directors were informed that individual student names were not collected for this study. A signed copy of the informed consent form can be viewed in Appendix B.

For the purpose of this qualitative study, and to maintain University of Phoenix participant anonymity, an identifier was created and assigned to each participant (Cantu, 2003; Neuman, 2003). An identifier was used for all 30 participants during data collection and data analysis, and was included as an eight-digit number representing the order in which the participant turned in the questionnaire. In order to follow the University of Phoenix's informed consent procedures, an alpha/numeric identifier was assigned (e.g., P1052209, P2052209) that identifies each participant, and the name was not revealed in this study. For clarity in discussing the participants' results in chapters 4 and 5, the participant identifiers were assigned a code name, such as Participant 1 and Participant 2 (see Appendix B). The questionnaires are retained in a safe place, with alpha/numeric identifiers to protect confidentiality. The questionnaires were stored in a locked file cabinet. All records containing the participants' information are retained for three years, after which the participants' information has to be destroyed (Warren & Karner, 2005).

Confidentiality

The participants were notified about the study being conducted in the community. The data from individuals for public health research must be balanced against individuals' rights to privacy and confidentiality, and should be based on human rights principles (UNAIDS, 2007). Thirty African American women were solicited for this study and were helpful with the outcomes of providing the research data. Leaders in the African American community were seen, as respectful, caring, and committed to community involvement. In order to attempt to counter the possibility that participants may feel obligated to participate in this study, two specific methods were included to insure informed consent was emphasized and understood. The participants received information listed on questionnaires about HIV/AIDS. The participants were informed about confidentiality. Permission to conduct this current study was granted by respectful community leaders and was reiterated to the participants (See Appendix B).

Validity

According to Heffner (2004), the reliability and validity of this qualitative, grounded theory study were based on the outcomes of the data to accurately and consistently represent attributes relating HIV/AIDS. In addition, the knowledge level of African American women helped to support the findings about this dreadful disease. Any conclusions regarding causation (internal validity) and generalization to other groups (external validity) were adequately controlled and disclosed. In fact, Heffner (2004), stated there are two basic forms of validity: (a) internal validity, where a researcher might infer a causal relationship or lack of a causal relationship between two variables; and (b) external validity, where a researcher may simplify the cause and effect relationship beyond the immediate subjects of the given study (Heffner, 2004).

Internal Validity

According to Heffner (2004), internal validity refers to the strength of conclusions drawn from a rigorous research design about theoretical information. Four sources of internal validity threats were reviewed with respect to this study, including (a) history, (b) maturation, (c) discovery, and (d) findings. Burden and Klofstad (2005), posits that although grounded theory retrospective designs do not allow the same degree of certainty as an experiment does, a well-designed grounded theory research study provides convincing theoretical evidence regarding the effects of one variable on another.

Variables other than the interventions under consideration were introduced between pre- and post-gathering of data, and may influence improvement in the qualitative results (Trochim, 2006). The factors, classified as history, may include unexpected answers from African American women (Burden & Klofstad, 2005). Thus, internal validity is only relevant in studies that try to establish a causal relationship, where the key question in internal validity is whether observed changes can be attributed to awareness (Trochim, 2006).

On the other hand, maturation was considered as a factor that might affect the results of the study. Improvement in data collection occurred as an intervention. African American women's awareness level about HIV/AIDS was investigated. This awareness level was not controlled in this study and was not disclosed as a limitation. Since the pre- and post-questionnaire designs were unknown at first, it was conceivable that the process of taking the questionnaire may affect the results. The questionnaire itself served as an intervention and actually helped to improve results on the post-questionnaire. A two-week interval between pre- and post-questionnaire helped control or influence the results. The participants were not informed that the questions were rearranged throughout the questionnaire to solicit the same or similar information in a different manner, which is asked in the pre-section of the questionnaire. According to Heffner (2004), the reliability of the questionnaires refers to the outcomes awareness results that were collected from the analyses. The validity of the questionnaires depended on the awareness levels of African American women. Both the validity and reliability of the qualitative, grounded theory questions were established through community college directors, and reported at the end of the study (Heffner, 2004).

External Validity

External validity refers to the ability to generalize about conclusions, regarding the theoretical results from the participant's awareness levels (Heffner, 2004). This current study was limited to an African American women population in two large cities (Dallas and Fort Worth, Texas). As a result, study findings were applicable to additional community college leaders.

Data Analysis

Reliability about HIV/AIDS awareness was assessed by reviewing the consistency of the questionnaire by line item and results (Eliot & Czarnolewski, 2007). The reliability of the questionnaire rested on the data results. Several authors note that the validity of an instrument refers to its suitability, significance, accuracy, and value of the inferences made from its scores (Turner, DeMers, Fox, & Reed, 2001). A valid questionnaire instrument measures what it was designed to measure correctly (Drain, 2004). To establish the validity of this questionnaire instrument, face validity and content validity were assessed by expert witnesses in their perspective specialties, such as health education, and community involvement (Palmquist, 2009). To validate the questionnaire data and theories, qualitative results were reported in this current study.

Distribution and collection of data was reported in four (4) stages. These stages provided the opportunity to reframe questions for the next round of five (5) participants after reading through and evaluating the earlier five questionnaires. The completion of the study would take approximately three weeks. The weeks would provide ample time to distribute, collect, and record the data results. In addition, the allowed time was used for studying and recording any late data that was received. The theoretical sampling is the process by which data was collected, coded and analyzed (Coleman & O'Connor, 2007). The initial sampling was the results of five participants. All the sets had eight alpha/numeric numbers and the process was in four (4) stages. Upon collection of the first set of data, assessments were made as to whether any questions for the next batch should be reframed. The ideas put forth in this set prompted another set of questions. An emerging core variable or theory was expected. The sources of data collection or the method of collecting data changed if necessary. Certain individuals may be interviewed for, further clarification of the data. The process of constant comparison continued until saturation or until no new data were possible.

Power (1996), MacLean and Mohr (1999) recommend several ways researchers can analyze the data that they have collected. The NVIVO coding of the collected data were recommended for collecting qualitative data. These codes were obtained from the participants questionnaires. Sorting was completed without interpretation. A large number of codes were emerged after the whole process was complete. Axial coding was used to relate categories to sub categories. Subsequently, selective coding, whereby the process of integration and refining the theory continued. Then, a process of recording the outcomes was monitored to provide theoretical results for the study.

Summary

The methodology selected for this current study was qualitative research that included the grounded theory design. The adopted methods proved important information. The research was iterative and emerging (Forman et al., 2008). The data were collected and studied each time a set of questions were collected, reviewed, and questions reframed as necessary. An emerging theory was seen at the end of the study (Tavakol, 2006). The emerging theory revealed that African American women did not know how to protect themselves from HIV/AIDS. The information gathered helped formulate innovative techniques for the population of African American women, who take the challenge of indulging in an intimate relationship. The knowledge gained from the peer education techniques initiated in this study, could save African American women with HIV/AIDS. The research analyses provided an acceptable degree of confidence, verification, and validation to maintain the accuracy, integrity, and consistency of the descriptive methods for this research (National Science Foundation, 2006). These analyses lead to a successful qualitative study. Finally, the results of the analyses, data coding, and questionnaires are explained in Chapter 4.

CHAPTER 4

RESULTS

This current study aimed at identifying factors that impact African American women and the lack of awareness about the HIV/AIDS disease. The alertness has become more frequent in the Dallas and Fort Worth areas of Texas. The willingness to communicate about HIV/AIDS has been a revelation. The participants used measures in terms of two hypotheses, namely: HIV/AIDS awareness and implications, which are different in African American women. HIV/AIDS has been recognized as an epidemic among African American women in the Dallas and Fort Worth areas of Texas, when discussing HIV/AIDS in the community. This chapter establishes a summary from the data collected from the participants. This discussion was followed by a detailed presentation of results that related to each of the two hypotheses. The hypotheses focused on the awareness about HIV/AIDS in regards to levels of intimate behavior. A summary of the main findings follow the hypotheses. In addition and where relevant, selected findings from the questionnaires were used to report any gaps and/or findings from the hypotheses. The final section of the chapter provides an overview of incidental findings relating to HIV/AIDS awareness.

Data Collection Procedures

A total of 30 college students currently enrolled in Dallas and Tarrant counties participated in this study. Of these, a total of 100 percent (corresponding to 30 students) were Africa American women. The women ranged from 18 to 54 years. Over 50 percent of the students participated from Dallas, another 50 percent were from Tarrant counties, and no other students are represented within this current study.

During data collection, participants were introduced to the symptoms of HIV for education purposes. In theory the affects of knowing some of the known symptoms, may prompt African American women to provide truthful answers to the questionnaire. In fact, the information would introduce them to a list of symptoms that would affect any woman with HIV/AIDS. Thus, encouraging them to answer truthfully and further validating the questionnaire results.

The AIDS symptoms that are listed within this research provide an overview of the hypotheses for this study. This information provides findings for symptoms of HIV/AIDS as well as the total number of valid responses (questionnaires) from each participant. An independent editor was selected to review the data to assure the raw data was entered into the master spreadsheet correctly. The data was checked for quality of the data transcription with a 100% review by the researcher to ensure quality data collection.

Symptoms of HIV/AIDS

All Health Network (2009) report that extreme fatigue; rapid weight loss from an unknown cause (more than 10 lbs. in two months for no reason); the appearance of swollen or tender glands in the neck, armpits or groin, for no apparent reason, lasting for more than four weeks; unexplained shortness of breath, frequently accompanied by a dry cough, not due to allergies or smoking; persistent diarrhea; intermittent high fever or soaking night sweats of unknown origin; a marked change in an illness pattern, either in frequency, severity, or length of sickness; the appearance of one or more purple spots on the surface of the skin, inside the mouth, anus or nasal passages; whitish coating on the tongue, throat or vagina; and forgetfulness, confusion and other signs of mental deterioration are known symptoms of HIV/AIDS (All Health Network, 2009). These symptoms are listed for informational purposes only, and not a substitute to diagnose or treat HIV/AIDS (Health Central, 2009).

Table 3

Participanst Results from Questionnaires: How will you save yourself from AIDS?

Participant Results from Questionnaires:	How will you save yourself from AIDS?
Dallas County Community College Participants	Tarrant County Community College Participants
P1060509 Abstinence, regular testing, protection	P16091109 Ask my doctor
P2060509 Protection and knowledge	P17091109 Be faithful and hope that my partner is too
P3060509 Practice safe sex	P18091109 Use condoms
P4060509 No answer provided	P19091109 No sex at all
P5060509 No answer provided	P20091109 No answer provided
P6060509 I don't know	P21091109 Abstinence
P7061209 Being without sex, safe sex	P22091109 Practice safe sex
P8061209 Trust that my husband is straight with me	P23091109 Communicate with my partner more
P9061209 Be protected, Information	P24091109 Use condoms
P10061209 Ask questions to have more knowledge	P25091109 Practice safe sex
P11061209 No sex at all, condoms, etc.	P26091109 Practice safe sex
P12061609 Stay married and pray for faithfulness	P27091109 Use condoms
P13061609 Don't mess around, protect myself	P28091109 Abstinence
P14061609 Not have blood transfusions, unprotect sex	P29091109 Use condoms
P15061609 Use protection, condoms	P30091109 Abstinence

Results from Study Hypotheses

As with any qualitative methodology, in grounded theory the researcher and the research design must remain flexible to account for emerging themes and patterns as the inquiry evolves (Glaser &

Strauss, 1967). Consistent with grounded theory methodology, the research was conducted using questionnaires with a random selection approach in which the data collection and analysis continued, until the sample size was reached (Strauss & Corbin, 1998). The results showed that community college students were willing to talk about HIV/AIDS awareness in the African American community. The awareness behaviors illustrated open-ended results and yielded answers from the structured questions. The following research question guided this study: (a) how will you save yourself from HIV/AIDS?"

The results from the hypotheses are illustrated in table three. The results show that the participants gained more knowledge about HIV/AIDS awareness.

1. Results from awareness levels: abstinence, being with the same partner (Dallas County P1-P15).
2. Results from awareness levels: learn more about HIV/AIDS, (Dallas County P1-P15).
3. Results from awareness levels: gain more knowledge about the disease, and get regular testing (Tarrant County P16-P30).
4. Results from awareness levels: communicate with partner, and abstinence (Tarrant County P16-P30).
5. Results from awareness levels: use condoms, practice safe sex, and abstinence (Tarrant County P16-P30).

Findings: Demographics

This research has uncovered important findings about awareness and African American women's perception about HIV/AIDS awareness and prevention. The results from the questionnaire provided direction for preventive measures, which is to contact a medical professional, community health leader, and read more data about prevention. The results from the study revealed a decision, as whether to implement individualized or community-based interventions for HIV/AIDS prevention. Two community colleges are included in the study. Dallas County Community College had 15 college students, and Tarrant County College had 15 students as well. The total of college students was 30, with a satisfied total return of all questionnaire results are included in the study.

Ethnicity and Gender in Community Colleges

The ethnicity breakdowns of African American participants in community college students are presented in Table 2. The percentages of college students were 50 percent from Dallas, and 50 percent from Tarrant Counties. There are no other ethnic groups included in this study. The questionnaires were distributed to community college students attending both Dallas and Tarrant Counties. The questionnaires were divided by ethnicity and gender (50 percent Dallas County African American women and 50 percent Tarrant County African American women). There were equal selections of the participants (15), although Dallas County had more African American community college students in attendance, than Tarrant County during the solicitation of the questionnaires.

Dallas County Community College Results

According to Freed (2006), the results from Dallas County have been reported according to the United Nations' AIDS epidemic report; more than 4 million people were infected with HIV in 2006. Almost 3 million people died due to AIDS in the same year. Since Acquired Immune Deficiency Syndrome was identified in 1981, more than 25 million people have passed away due to AIDS-related causes. An entire generation of smart, talented, and creative people has died from the disease (Freed, 2006). The Dallas County results have benefited the students as a step towards improving the health in the communities (Schenker & Nyirenda, 2002).

Tarrant County College Results

Tarrant County and the AIDS Outreach Center (2007) reported that several accomplishments have resulted from the AIDS Outreach Center (AOC). The AIDS Outreach Center stands alone as the lead HIV/AIDS agency and the major point of outreach, testing, and education in the seven county areas of North Central Texas (AOC, 2007). A goal was to aggressively educate the general population about behavioral risks associated with HIV infection, identify target populations already at-risk for HIV infection, and to bring those already infected with HIV into the

AOC for medical care and treatment services program to assure access to quality of life and medical care services (AOC, 2007).

The AOC (2007) results illustrated, the 2008-2009 fiscal years were successful despite the downturn in the local, state, and national economies. While funding appeals to communities of faith, fraternal/social/community organizations, local business, and national corporations has seen increases of as much as 800 percent over the last fiscal year. Annual giving from individuals and foundations has dropped (AOC, 2007).

Findings: African American women share a Sense of Urgency

Major Theme One—Part A

African American women report that not enough education about HIV/AIDS was supported through leadership. They express a sense of urgency for their communities and people they know. African American women are concerned about more education, because they do not want their children infected with HIV/AIDS. A majority of American women have been tested for HIV; why have two out of five African American women (40 percent) not been tested for HIV (Kaiser Family Foundation, 1998).

Major Theme One—Part B

African American women are concerned about becoming infected. Almost half, (46 percent) say that AIDS is a more urgent problem today for their local community than it was a few years ago. A majority (55 percent) of African American women say that AIDS is a serious problem for people they know; and 50 percent know someone personally who has AIDS, has died of AIDS, or has tested positive for HIV (Kaiser Family Foundation, 1998).

Major Theme Two

Theme two describes HIV/AIDS and Relative Racial Distributions of people diagnosed with HIV/AIDS. Figure 1 shows the results from different races the communities. The results illustrate a comparison of different races in regards to people diagnosed with HIV/AID (CDC, 2004). As the impact of HIV/AIDS on African Americans has grown over time, so have the Centers for Disease Control and Prevention's (CDC) efforts to address it. The CDC has been committed to reducing the disparities that exist among African Americans, but the agency has come to realize that it cannot take on such an enormous task alone. The CDC believes that a heightened, urgent, and collaborative response among the CDC, community members, and influential leaders is necessary to decrease HIV/AIDS among African Americans (CDC, 2004). For instance, African Americans in general, believe that AIDS is a more urgent problem for their local community and a problem that some leaders do not have enough knowledge about, and/or willing to speak about publicly, because of the stigma associated with the disease (Kaiser Family Foundation, 1998).

Major Theme Three

African Americans support federal spending on HIV/AIDS. African Americans show support for more government efforts in the fight against AIDS. Most believe that the government is not spending enough money on AIDS (66 percent). Even when compared to the amount of money the federal government spends on other health problems, such as heart disease or cancer, a majority (54 percent) still say spending on AIDS is too low. The support of African Americans for spending not only stands out above that of all other Americans (40 percent says the federal government spending is too low in the context of other health problems) but also has endured over time. In 1995, 58 percent said spending was too low, even in light of spending on other health problems (Kaiser Family Foundation, 1998).

Major Theme Four

Theme four encompasses Community College Students' knowledge about HIV/AIDS in Texas. Community college students understand how they can prevent the transmission of HIV but are less knowledgeable about HIV/AIDS testing (RedOrbit.com, 2008). Addressing the health needs (knowledge about HIV/AIDS) of college students is replete with unique challenges. Most have yet to confront ethics, respect for their own bodies, mortality, and illness, which was seen as an unfortunate stroke of fate that befalls others. Luquis, Garcia, and Ashford (2003) report that college students' perception of health is that it is not a major concern, because they are young, vibrant, knowledgeable, and we have condoms to protect us. Most respondents defined health as not having any known disease, mental or physical problems.

Most college students were not concerned about the disease. When asked how concerned they were about health, most college students responded that they were not concerned about the disease. When the same students were asked about HIV/AIDS and the effects of the dreaded disease in the African American community, the majority viewed it as common among peers, with estimates of 80-90 percent of students using some type of (health prevention). The methods identified were abstinence, regular testing, and protection. Results also indicated that sexual experimentation was not only part of college, but also it was expected (Biscaro, 2004).

Interventions

Findings: Interpretations

This research reports one way to attract attention to African American women and an attempt to provide awareness about HIV/AIDS prevention. In order to attempt to prevent African American women from infection of HIV/AIDS, appropriate preventive interventions were required. The risk and problem behavioral results shown on the questionnaire suggest different approaches to such interventions. For HIV/AIDS prevention to increase among African American women, both the African American community programs and resources about awareness issues should be addressed. The Centers for Disease Control and Prevention has developed an HIV intervention called *Street Smart* that has been proven effective among communities in the U.S. If *Street Smart* were implemented in the Dallas/Fort Worth community colleges, it could increase HIV/

AIDS awareness and possibly reduce chances of contracting HIV/ AIDS (Centers for Disease Control and Prevention, 2007).

The results of this study contribute to effective interventions. Appendix C illustrates the present study results. There were no contradictory findings among the community college participants. It was expected that the questionnaire would have an overall positive effect on the women, in terms of increased positive awareness about HIVAIDS. The findings presented by the questionnaire showed that the anticipated results were not only expected, but also rather showed more of an opportunity to implement new HIV/AIDS awareness strategies, such as the ones mentioned within this research. By providing structured, open-ended questions, the results showed that the questionnaire yielded favorable results from the African American women. With the use of the questionnaire, the participants could look at the progress of their knowledge levels over time and revisit whether or not their results changed. The progression of HIV/AIDS information could encourage these women to become motivated to view awareness about HIV/AIDS as a positive prevention. The results revealed that their knowledge levels increased in awareness about HIV/AIDS.

Significance to the Responses

The results indicated that the hypotheses in the present study were based soundly on previous research and theory. The inconsistency and relative lack of information provided by the questionnaire results, as well as the fact that African American women did not know what specific questions would be asked, posed limits to the study. Since, they did not have the questions beforehand; suggest that perhaps there were certain limitations to the study, such as definitions to some of the words and terms indicated on the questionnaire. The use of strike-through questions in the present study introduced unanticipated results. These unanswered questions could have provided detailed information in reporting the findings of the study.

For the participants, they may not have known the answers to some of the terms, thereby leaving a gap in the questionnaire results. This gap was alleviated by providing answers to questions, such as definitions and reading the questions to the participants, in order to help gain a better understanding of the questionnaires. They had some hesitation about revealing private information in this qualitative grounded-theory study. This factor is important not only to the data analysis of the present study, but also to the question of applicability of the results to the use of truth telling when taking a doctoral research questionnaire.

Specifically, the research methods were explained in detail to reassure the participants that all information would be held confidential. No one would have any way of knowing who provided the intimate information, because each of the participants were assigned a participant non-identifiable code (e.g., P1061509). The information was provided in plain white envelopes upon distribution. Upon collection of the packets, the participants were instructed to seal the envelopes, and return the packets to a designated box. They were given a chance to place their individual packets within the stack of previously collected envelopes, so that the researcher would not have any chance of identifying the participant, thus protecting the participants' identity.

Outlier: Unanswered Questions

While the previously mentioned theories offer insight into the knowledge and awareness about HIV/AIDS. Some important questions remain unanswered. Presumptions were made based on ideas that African American women would vary in their levels of knowledge, awareness, and intelligence in regards to this study. The difference in the responses made it unclear whether diversity played a role as an advantage or disadvantage to answering questions on the questionnaire. The results and ideas were uncertain as to whether a differentiation exists between non degreed in opposition to potential degreed community college students. Some points to ponder are as follows: College students that have completed most of their courses at a community college have an educational advantage over those who are entry-level community college students, when answering research questions about awareness of HIV/AIDS.

Ethnic and gender concerns were noted as an issue of the levels of HIV/AIDS awareness. The investigation about awareness had interesting implications from both the Dallas and Fort Worth college students that were involved in the study. Due to research studies pertaining to levels of awareness, community leaders and activist have been advised about the effects of HIV/AIDS awareness. The leaders are now researching, studying, asking questions, and attending government sponsored classes to become better equipped to deal with the community affected by HIV/AIDS (CDC, 2004).

According to Dunham (2007), socio-demographic variables including ethnicity, age, and gender have an important impact on HIV/AIDS awareness in the community. African Americans around the nation are disproportionately impacted by HIV/AIDS (Dunham, 2007). This study revealed efforts that addressed the disparity and identified meaningful interventions to reduce HIV/AIDS among African Americans. This current study provided participants with the opportunity to voice their concerns about the rising HIV/AIDS epidemic in the African American community. This study facilitated the epidemiological revelations of (30) voices, from the Dallas/Fort Worth areas of Texas, that were able to speak out about the need for alliances and potential partnerships that mutually enhanced the capacity to build effective HIV/AIDS prevention and care strategies.

Strength of the Study

Despite probable limitations, this current study possesses several strengths. This study may be the first of its kind to reveal results about an awareness level of HIV/AIDS from African American women in Dallas and Fort Worth, Texas. The strength, validity, privacy, and outcomes have proved valuable to the participants, by providing awareness about HIV/AIDS. The participants were happy to be able to gain knowledge, while learning from the questionnaire. The use of gathering succinct information from college students has gained immense popularity over the past twenty years. It is important to remember that college students want to express their opinions and have their voices heard in the community (SinoFresh HealthCare, 2009).

Summary

Perceived awareness behaviors from community college students were an emergent result from the research. By their own account, the results affected their knowledge levels and willingness to talk about HIV/AIDS awareness. The findings from the questionnaire supported the hypotheses. The results show that concerns for education, training, and abstinence are concerns in regards to HIV/AIDS awareness.

The results showed concern from the participants, as they became aware of the information on the questionnaire. Beginning of the July 2009, 30 questionnaires were completed for this research. The results from the questionnaires revealed the effects of awareness of the disease. Appendix B described the informed consent information, which allowed the participants to volunteer to give intimate information about HIV/AIDS. The information was used to analyze the data in order to search for differences in the qualitative data at the time of the awareness intervention. Each participant's results were entered into a Microsoft Excel database to review the overall results, and record the information into an omniscient narrative form.

CHAPTER 5

CONCLUSIONS AND RECOMMENDATIONS

The results of this current study yielded practical data about HIV/AIDS awareness from African American women. The study produced data about how socio-economic status affected the risk of contracting HIV/AIDS, and the nature and extent of the fatal disease on African American women attending community colleges (CDC, 2006). CDC (2006) states that most women with some awareness of HIV/AIDS were not expected to contract the HIV/AIDS disease. According to the CDC (2006), receiving more education, knowledge, and training theoretically offered a better chance of not contracting the disease in the African American community. Lack of awareness of the HIV/AIDS disease placed women in a crisis, as high risk for an AIDS-related illness or death (CDC, 2006). Misconception was the most common in Terminal cases. The survey responses revealed that some African American women knew about the possible outcomes, but did not respond seriously to preventative measures.

The Importance of Who Cares

One of the goals of the Centers for Disease Control and Prevention is African American women are aware of the consequences of contracting the HIV/AIDS disease (CDC, 2003). Community initiatives and education interventions have been established across the United States in an attempt to meet the demand for HIV/ AIDS prevention (CDC, 2007). Despite billions of federal dollars spent on closing the awareness gap, there is still a lack in this area among African American women when compared to other races (CDC, 2004). The Centers for Disease Control and Prevention (2008) reported that African American women are not taking the initiative to get published information about HIV/AIDS awareness and prevention. This research illustrates a qualitative, grounded theory study, which reveals information about the lack of awareness of HIV/AIDS. The study aims to assess the state of awareness of HIV/AIDS among African American women, and improve on that awareness. Data was collected from the Dallas/Fort Worth areas of Texas on 30 African American women's lack of awareness about the HIV/AIDS threat to the community, the stigma associated with HIV/ AIDS, and the burden incurred by families when African American women die from this disease. Fears related to disclosure and stigmas were frequently reported than were fears of dying of HIV/AIDS. Limitations were financial, sexual/reproductive, and physical. Physical limitations were related to the presence of symptoms leading to a wide range of emotions (Jackson-Gray, 1999). The researcher explored the implications of these research study findings, which influenced African American women to read data and consider the possible outcomes of contracting HIV/AIDS (Avert, 2009). The research methods applied to this study included questionnaires that were analyzed line-by-line using NVIVO coding processes.

Information Not Reported

This current HIV/AIDS research does not investigate into the ways in which the disease completely overturns the life of an infected person (Okechukwu, 2009). The grief of those who have contracted the virus is so devastating that the information has not been accurately reported (CDC, 2003), as such exposure would scare the American population. The pictures of infected women would put Americans on alarm about the disease and cause a true panic; placing the information on television, radio, and in the media on a daily, weekly, and monthly basis would cause uproar in American communities (Culshaw, 2006). The information about HIV/AIDS is mostly found in written format, which places some people at a disadvantage, as they are unprepared or unable to gain access to the information (Kiyaga, 2008). Rarely does anyone talk about the grief, anger, pride, shame, and stigma on a collective basis. AIDS education may help to diminish the stigmas associated with the HIV/AIDS disease. These obstructions to awareness and prevention can cause grief and, in association with this grief, great anger (CDC Business Labor Resource Service, 1992).

Grief Experience

Goldblum and Erickson (2000) have identified facets of grief. These facets are grief response, which is the grief of continuing to dwell on the person who may have transmitted the HIV/AIDS disease to the infected party; the state of the infected party's medical and financial affairs; a need to think repeatedly about past events; a sense of guilt; even thoughts of suicide. As Goldblum and Erickson (2000) state, the grief experience never goes away; those infected with HIV/AIDS continue to grieve until they die (Goldblum & Erickson, 2000).

Effective grief/distress interventions range from educational activities to psychotherapy. The information listed within this chapter describes activities and methods for matching grieving activities to mourners as needed. Table 4 lists a psychotherapeutic approach with Integrative AIDS Grief/Distress Relief Therapy that combines aspects of psychodynamic and cognitive behavioral therap. The approach enhances recent developments specifically designed to assist AIDS mourners in reducing the risk of complicated grief, anger, and mourning (Goldblum & Erickson, 2000).

Communities vary in terms of which services are available for AIDS mourners. To some degree, the extent of services is consistent with the magnitude of the problem. The communities hit the hardest by the epidemic, especially those in the Dallas and Fort Worth areas of Texas; have established the most extensive support systems. Goldblum and Erickson (2000) state that the first step is for leaders and clinicians to determine the types of services available in their communities; once this resource map is constructed, clinicians can match mourners to appropriate grief/distress relief interventions based on the individualized assessment described in this chapter. While a discussion of community-wide health planning is outside the scope of this study, it is important to note that the selection of AIDS grief interventions described in Table 4 could be useful in designing a community-wide response to this problem (Goldblum & Erickson, 2000).

Table 4

Level of Grief/Distress and Potential Interventions

Level of Grief/Distress   Grief/Distress Relief Interventions

One: Uncomplicated mourning without risk factors	AIDS Grief Education and Support Community Support Classes			
Two: Uncomplicated Mourning with Risk Factors	AIDS Grief Education and Support Community Support Classes	Grief/ Distress & Relief Risk Reduction Counseling		
Three: Complicated Mourning without Clinical Disorder	AIDS Grief Education and Support Community Support Classes	Grief/ Distress & Relief Risk Reduction Counseling	Grief-Related Psychotherapy	
Four: Complicated Mourning with Clinical Disorder	AIDS Grief Education and Support Community Support Classes	Grief/ Distress & Relief Risk Reduction Counseling	Grief-Related Psychotherapy	Psychiatric Evaluation and Treatment

Note. Adapted from Goldblum & Erickson, 2000.

Pride in Dealing with Illnesses and Diseases

Goldblum and Erickson (2000) advocate for illness and disease awareness and prevention. There was a phrase used: "smile with pride." This phrase was implemented to encourage those affected by and illness or disease to do their part to end the stigma associated with the disease. Goldblum and Erickson (2000) describe how urban renewal policies from the 1940s through the 1960s destroyed poor, communities, tearing apart social bonds and leaving the inhabitants vulnerable to the spread of heroin, crack, and AIDS. They show how a combination of factors including what might have been the intentional abandonment of those affected by poverty. Goldblum and Erickson (2000) present a close look inside the minds of the people involved, revealing how, in the aftermath of this outbreak of disease, fear, cultural ignorance, pride, homophobia, and even love worked together to stigmatize HIV/AIDS and ultimately made it harder to study, prevent, and treat the disease in the African American community. Moreover, Goldblum and Erickson (2000) detail how the initial identification of the disease as a "gay disease" ultimately pitted the white gay community against the African American community in the battle for public health funding (Goldblum & Erickson, 2000).

Who Gets AIDS

The American Heritage Dictionary (2009) defines the word *stigma* as a mark of disgrace or infamy, a stain or reproach, as on a person's reputation (Minge, 2008). The HIV/AIDS disease affects everyone in the United States: African Americans, Arab Americans, Asian, Pacific Americans, disabled people, gay men, Native Americans, older peoples, prisoners, sex workers, healthcare workers, sexual abuse victims, hemophiliacs, substance abusers, heterosexual men, suburban and rural populations, the homeless, transgendered people, immigrants, U.S. military personnel, Latinos and Latinas, women, lesbians, and young people (The Body: The Complete HIV/AIDS Resource, 2010). Due to stigmatization, HIV related grief awareness has not been recognized or validated by society. Responses to the issue of mandatory AIDS testing, for example, have not protested the possible human rights violations such testing involves. Testing without permission is an invasion of privacy and contributed to stigmas.

A Leadership Perspective

African Americans have called on all levels of leadership for HIV/AIDS awareness and prevention. The U.S. government has been the world leader in responding to the global pandemic of HIV/AIDS, and has made the fight against HIV/AIDS a top priority. This top priority issue represents everyone; not only, for humanitarian reasons, but for the HIV/AIDS crisis which threatens the prosperity, stability, and development of nations around the world (USAID, 2009).

Bishop, T. D. Jakes

The Black Christian community has been instrumental in acting on their own, and recruiting government aid, in the fight against HIV/AIDS. HIV/AIDS education provided by the leaders of the federal government focuses on prevention, testing, treatment, research, and the use of new media in response to HIV/AIDS (AIDS. gov, 2009). A collective of black church leaders have called upon the U.S. Government to declare an HIV/AIDS crisis in the African American community. A public health emergency and the recent conclave, hosted by The National Black Leadership Commission on AIDS, marked the first time African American leaders from all sectors, including clergy, scholars, government, and health agencies, convened to develop a plan for ending HIV/AIDS in black America. Prominent black ministers, including mega church pastor Bishop T. D. Jakes of The Potter's House, Dallas, Texas, pledged that the church would play its role in bringing awareness and promoting testing of HIV/AIDS to the faith community (Phan, 2007).

Nelson Mandela

Leaders from around the world have come together to solve conflicts in dealing with HIV/AIDS and the stigma associated with the disease. The program Eminent Persons Ecumenical Program for

Africa (EPEPA) launched the names of prominent leaders serving as members of the traveling task force to become the speakers for the world at large on behalf of HIV/AIDS issues. The list of more than 25 names included former South African President Nelson Mandela, Bishop Desmond Tutu, and Nobel Laureate Wangari Maathai of Kenya (Vu, 2005). The African peace program relies on the incredible resource embodied in the elders and distinguished individuals already in our midst. It is the duty of these leaders to resolve conflicts in communities in Africa, said the Rev. John McCullough, executive director and CEO of Church World Service (CWS): The moral authorities, of these wise and renowned eminent Africans Americans have helped to bring leaders to the table to negotiate peace (Vu, 2005).

The program was developed out of the awareness of the faith community's history of successfully promoting peaceful relations among African Americans, as well as a desire to be more aggressive about intervening at a reconciling presence to stop the widespread violence on the continent (Vu, 2005). The agency has intensified work in resolving HIV/AIDS and peace building in Africa and throughout the world. Specifically, Mandela announced the death of his son due to AIDS-related complications, hoping that such openness might contribute to awareness and the fight of the stigma of AIDS (Vu, 2005).

President Barack Obama

The President acknowledged the importance of the struggle against HIV/AIDS while still a senator. During his speech to a crowd of nearly 10,000 people, Obama, a member of Trinity UCC in Chicago, criticized division within the church, but praised Christian leaders and groups that have worked together to remedy social problems. "That's why pastors, friends of mine like Rick Warren and T.D. Jakes and organizations like World Vision and Catholic Charities are wielding their enormous influence to confront poverty, HIV/AIDS, and the genocide in Darfur," Obama said (Vu, 2007).

Obama has also spoken about strong political and governmental commitment of leadership at all levels that can translate into real actions and support, which is necessary for sustained and effective interventions against HIV/AIDS epidemic. There is huge potential for spiritual and socio-cultural values and opportunities to become integrated with proven scientific knowledge; politicians, government, such as President Barack Obama, along with religious leaders and faith-based organizational groups could play a leading role in the fight against HIV/AIDS.

The Church Cares about HIV/AIDS

The church, as a known safe haven for all, is active in the fight against HIV/AIDS. When a person contracts the HIV virus or AIDS, they often call for prayer from a local, community church. Churches have to be prepared to pray with and/or for, counsel, listen, and provide community outreach support to those who are struggling with HIV/AIDS (Kwon, 2007).

Many diseases that plague humankind are not preventable; this is not the case with HIV/AIDS, where awareness and education can be hugely instrumental in thwarting the disease. There are those who, as a result, may hold those who suffer from AIDS accountable for contracting HIV in the first place, but the church promotes awareness rather than blame. Moreover, millions of women receive the disease from unfaithful husbands, millions of babies are born to HIV positive mothers, and millions become HIV positive through tainted blood supplies (Kwon, 2007).

The church leaders work in every capacity, cooperatively with communities and hospitals, in response to the global HIV/AIDS epidemic. African Americans go to church to seek care for orphans and those who are dying of AIDS. One goal of church leadership has been to teach abstinence, which has reduced the HIV/AIDS crisis (Population Services International, 2009). The church accommodates families affected by HIV/AIDS (Kwon, 2007).

Benefits from the HIV/AIDS Research

Yu, Souteyrand, Banda, Kaufman, and Perriens (2008) reported there is increasing debate regarding whether investment in HIV/AIDS research and intervention programs is strengthening or weakening the U.S. health system. Their study examined access, evidence, and initiatives, and, based off the results, proposed ways to present a level of awareness to the global society about the benefits from HIV/AIDS research. Together with global initiative, the African American communities and health systems must prepare to become client-perspective based on systems oriented towards both awareness and prevention of the HIV/AIDS disease.

The study reported that major Global Health Initiatives have implemented awareness programs in countries with widespread HIV/AIDS problems. Among the positive impacts have been the increased awareness of, and priority given to, public health by governments. Services for those living with HIV/AIDS have rapidly expanded. Throughout the world, the infrastructure and laboratories have been strengthened; and in some cases, primary health care services have been improved (Yu et al., 2008). The effect of AIDS on the health workforce has been lessened by the provision of antiretroviral treatment to HIV infected health care workers, by training, and to an extent, by task shifting. There are reports of concerns about increasing AIDS funding and stagnant reproductive health funding, and accusations that workers from health care services are offered better-paying jobs in HIV/AIDS programs. Unfortunately, there is limited hard evidence of these claims (Harries, Maher, & Nunn, 1997).

Service delivery for AIDS has not reached a level that could conceivably be considered, as close to global access as possible (Harries et al., 1997). Countries and development partners must maintain the momentum of investment in HIV/AIDS awareness and preventive programs. The global action for healthcare has been more underfunded than the response to the HIV epidemic. The real issue has not been noted as whether to fund AIDS or health systems; but how to increase funding altogether (Yu et al., 2008).

The evidence from this research supported the previous consensus regarding the impact of HIV/AIDS on health systems and the debate about who benefits from the HIV/AIDS research: primarily, global health partnerships. Current information about responses to HIV/AIDS could be maintained and strengthened to benefit awareness approaches. Instead of endless debates about the comparative advantages of vertical and horizontal approaches, health systems and partners should focus on the best use for investments in strengthening the primary health care systems in an attempt to decrease the spread of HIV/AIDS (Yu et al., 2008).

The Reactions about Awareness

There are two primary ways to react to the information in this current HIV/AIDS research. Community health foundations should verify that the information is accurate. Health care providers working within HIV-oriented organizations should disseminate information on HIV/AIDS research studies, services and information regarding HIV/AIDS treatments, prevention, testing, risk factors, research, and clinical trials (San Francisco AIDS Foundation, 2009). They can be part of the effort to increase awareness, which, as evidence demonstrates, leads to positive results.

First, an accurate source of information on HIV/STD education, referrals, and support for over 90 years should be reviewed and placed on alert for all communities affected by this disease. The American Social Health Administration (ASHA) mission should be implemented as a preventive measure to help stop sexually transmitted diseases and their effects (American Social Health Association, 2009). A comprehensive AIDS information service, with accurate and timely information for everyone, is vital in enabling people to combat the AIDS epidemic, (U.S. National Library of Medicine, 2009).

A key element in designing and implementing service delivery programs for HIV/AIDS is the evaluation and global watch of those programs that already disseminate information. The Internet is an excellent way to reach a large audience, and HIV/AIDS programs make good use of the information. A selection of materials for evaluating direct services, as well as training programs focused on HIV/AIDS, could be provided in a range of formats, such as standardized tests, self-administered questionnaires, structured interviews, guidelines for qualitative data collection, and other methods. Both quantitative and qualitative evaluation approaches could be represented (Avert, 2009). Additionally, major university studies, governmental agencies, and countries around the world could have access to useable information. Large computer systems (domains) could list HIV/AIDS information as advertisement to solicit hits each month. The rate at which new users access websites could provide pertinent information that the federal government may be able to use as an intervention tool.

Websites such as MySpace, Facebook, and YouTube could be used as pilot programs to spread the news about HIV/AIDS awareness. In this way, lessons could be extended to those who may be aware of the effects of HIV/AIDS. Solicitation pop-ups could be placed on many other websites to either slow down or even eliminate harsh traffic. Because there is so much traffic to these websites, many users throughout the world would become informed, and this new innovative model of HIV/AIDS services would spread to a worldwide audience. Thus, a goal of awareness would meet the needs of the community, and the results would yield effective means and goals for data collection, with widely disseminated information about HIV/AIDS (Huba et al., 1998).

Attitude Functions

The final section of this research provides an overview of incidental findings relating to attitude functions about HIV/AIDS. A total of 30 participants from the Dallas and Fort Worth areas of Texas participated in this study. Incidental findings from the study illustrated that some participants were not supportive in their attitudes when talking about HIV/AIDS, and that some community college students do not believe that social norms and education are important. College students who have a high level of perceived behavioral control would be prone to address issues about HIV/AIDS with those in their families. The overall incidental model for using attitudes, social norms and educational controls would predict future community college students' intentions to talk about HIV/AIDS. Attitudes emerge only as a conversation topic, however, when comparing community college students with high consistent future intentions with community college students who have no intention to talk about HIV/AIDS.

As stated in Chapter 1, this current study results identify factors that affect the level of awareness about HIV/AIDS. Willingness to communicate about HIV/AIDS has been in evidence, judging by the responses to the questionnaire. There was some evidence from the questionnaire that community college students struggle with the fact that it is not immediately apparent to them about how a person can get HIV/AIDS. Simply put, prejudice and discrimination can be directed at those who only talk about HIV/AIDS, and even more so towards those who conduct research with community college students and their associated communities. Talking about HIV/AIDS can result in people being rejected by their families, from their community, shunned, discriminated against, or even physically hurt (Avert, 2009).

Importance of Research

The important thing to know about the HIV/AIDS research is how to stay HIV negative. This research was designed with a general disclaimer that was intended to inform the reader about levels of awareness about HIV/AIDS and African American women. This research study was designed for educational purposes, and not presented to engage in rendering medical advice or professional services to the readers. The information has been provided through the University of Phoenix, School of Academic Studies Doctoral Program for research purposes only. The research methods that may be listed or eluded to should not be used for diagnosing or treating a health problem or a disease. They are not a substitute for professional care. If one has or suspects that one may have HIV and/or AIDS, they should consult a health care provider (Bell, 1998).

The AIDS pandemic has already resulted in the deaths of approximately 11.7 million people worldwide (Bell, 1998). HIV has ultimately caused the deaths of an estimated 30.6 million men, women, and children around the globe still living with this disease. Roughly, 6 million people were newly infected with HIV in 1997; and nearly 16,000 more people die each day from this devastating disease (Bell, 1998).

Implications

This section provides evidence that awareness about HIV/AIDS have an important impact on those in the African American community. This section analyzed examples of awareness among community college students, specifically those not aware of the outcomes of the disease. When leaders, who serve as informants or policy-makers deal with Human Immunodeficiency Virus/ Acquired Immunodeficiency Syndrome (HIV/AIDS) problems about awareness will arise. The need for a community and/or social response as the public realizes the severe need for awareness about HIV/AIDS has become a main concern for African American women. A theoretical framework was developed and applied in the form of a questionnaire to solicit community results from participants. These two groups were from the local community colleges and were used in engaging with HIV/AIDS awareness results.

The implications of these results were combined with the results of how women identified themselves in relation to such outcomes in the areas of the HIV/AIDS disease. Random House Dictionary (2009) reports that an implication was defined as the relation that holds between two propositions, or classes of propositions, in virtue of which one was logically deducible from the other (Random House Dictionary, 2009); the question of whether definitions have any impact on action was examined. The section provided a useful grounded theory, theoretical framework based on awareness that links HIV/AIDS awareness at the local and international levels.

Implications for Leadership

The main implication for leadership in this current study is the need to address and heighten awareness about crucial aspects in the fight against HIV/AIDS, producing a political approach where leadership, adequate resources, and multi-sectoral approaches are recognized (United Nations Economic Commission for Africa and UNAIDS, 2003). The AIDS epidemic has undermined the foundation of economic development and the possibilities of its long-term sustainability in Texas; an integrated effort at all levels of leadership was needed to counter this damage and to avoid its further spread. Serious political commitment and adequate resource allocation are essential elements in saving the lives of millions of people and the economic viability of the societies involved. In addition, more knowledge was needed about the complex interactions of various factors and how they affect the spread of the epidemic, in order to develop appropriate prevention initiatives. AIDS issues could be addressed through any single factor in isolation, but must be brought into our neighborhoods and communities for a more comprehensive approach.

Community leaders can get involved in HIV/AIDS awareness. This leadership stage could be implemented on a state level, on a civil or social level, via NGOs, religious and social leaders, community and opinion leaders, and the academic community as well. This would create a strong, effective and sustained national and international leadership effort that would be able to promote a better understanding of awareness. This level of awareness could spread among leaders at all levels, ensuring a political commitment to combating AIDS; creating awareness of the processional nature of leadership; ensuring global health policy; and developing appropriate awareness indicators for the monitoring and evaluation of HIV/AIDS interventions. Leaders would need additional training about sensitive information that supported economic means and operational tools to implement these education and advocacy goals for a change in HIV/AIDS awareness. Leaders could make a positive difference in the communities (Loewenson, 2001).

Researcher Surprises

As stated in Chapter 1, awareness was the focus of this current study, and the most startling of the research results was the participant's completion of intimate, private, invasive, and research study without hesitation. Women of other races wanted to complete the questionnaire, but they were informed that only a specific population could be included in the research, so that the results would not be skewed. The reasons behind the parameters were explained succinctly, and the participants understood the protocol for the research. There was a concern that the community college students might have become discouraged or even resentful towards the study as they read the intimate questions. They were assured that the responses on the questionnaires would be kept confidential and would help other African American women in regards to awareness about HIV/AIDS, and possibly prevent other women from contracting HIV/AIDS. The women were excited and anxious about filling out the questionnaire; one community college student commented specifically on the fact that students would be able to learn important information from the provisions of the questionnaire (see Table 3).

Recommendations

The researcher recommends that an awareness model should be developed, and implemented by leaders in the community. A model provided by the National HIV/AIDS Elimination Act would provided some steps for communication between leaders, activists, HIV/AIDS patients, and those who are HIV negative. These leaders could conduct awareness meetings, protecting the privacy of those involved, and provide data protection assessments that would ensure that the provisions of all are followed on a local, state, and federal basis. The development of such a model should build on existing practices and experiences gained in community outreach programs. HIV/AIDS programs are recommended, to further lessen the gaps in knowledge about HIV/AIDS. By facilitating dialogue and cooperation among the leaders in the community, this recommendation represents the prime example in privacy, confidentiality, and awareness of the rights of all who may participate in and/or benefit from HIV/AIDS awareness. For the purposes of the protection of personal data, research and development, it is recommended that leaders should cooperate with other community representatives, researchers, doctoral learners, state and local governments, and those in support of HIV/AIDS research and awareness, in order to stimulate and support the introduction of the HIV/AIDS awareness in the African American community. This recommendation allows the research design to become effective at all levels of the community. Leaders should take all necessary measures to bring this recommendation to the attention of anyone with stakes in the design and operation of HIV/AIDS awareness initiatives within a community.

The results from the questionnaires indicate that the leaders in the communities should work with outreach programs to maintain a local advocacy program in Texas. The emphasis should be placed on awareness and resource commitments. Awareness opportunities should be taken into account to advocate a gendered response, and promote a successful technique of collaborating and learning about development programs on HIV/AIDS.

The leaders should work with representatives and sponsors to develop a strategy for promoting evaluation questionnaires and research into the impact of the disease at the local, national, and regional levels. Priority should be given to results revealing behavioral change and related factors, including gender, stigma, and poverty. The implementation of community models could produce awareness conventions on HIV/AIDS (arranged by the representatives and sponsors), which should be continued and expanded to reflect all disease-levels as well. This recommendation could lend itself as a research model in order to increase awareness and decrease the possibility of contracting HIV/AIDS.

Future Research

The importance of future research could be used for governmental use, and a more comprehensive view of the results from this research. The information would be helpful in improving the quality of information available to African American women, and would enable leaders to interact in support of the participant's responses. Understanding the challenge of providing awareness would be useful to future researchers seeking to expound on the attitudes and stigma associated with HIV/AIDS. As noted, awareness, behavior, and stigma may be a challenge for future researchers, who are overshadowed by the potential benefits of this research. The results of this current study should not be a reason for procrastination in future research studies (Simon, 2006). Future researchers could profit and expand on levels of awareness by including a larger sampling, of more than 30 African American women in future research.

Summary

The intent of this research was achieved by answering the research question revealing how African American women anticipated saving themselves from HIV/AIDS. This current study demonstrated that individual awareness levels among college students influence their willingness to talk about HIV/AIDS awareness. By distinguishing between the different hypotheses, this study suggests that individual awareness levels (such as personal knowledge, education, and training about HIV/AIDS) consistently influenced all students' answers. The answers from the results may ultimately become a major objective of leaders in the communities as a way to improve HIV/AIDS awareness. Improving awareness may be a difficult task; however, it is the duty and responsibility of everyone. This duty requires a meaningful change in the way leaders cooperate on a community level. This transition would require leaders to communicate at a different structural level, and increase awareness and prevention, about HIV/AIDS (CDC, 2003).

This study assessed the awareness levels of HIV/AIDS participants among African American women. As stated in Appendix D, community college students were used as participants to examine African American women's lack of awareness about the HIV/AIDS. The researcher explored the implications of the study findings, and the potential to influence African American women to read data that are more public and consider the possible outcomes of contracting HIV/AIDS. Key findings from the results have revealed that the awareness intervention model was successful in raising awareness in the selected population.

Conclusion

This study presented examples, detailed information, and emerging theory about HIV/AIDS awareness (WHO, 2005). For this current study, data was collected from 30 community college students representing Dallas and Fort Worth, Texas, between the ages of 18-54 years. Chapter 4 describes the data collection, results, demographic breakdown, and data analyses processes.

Some examples of literature are listed from around the world for the years 1967 to 2010 to support findings for Texas. Detailed information was collected from African American women who attend community colleges, and information was collected from questionnaires given to these community college students in Dallas and Fort Worth, Texas. This research does not include those students, from other races, or those who are not in attendance at areas listed in this research (Centers for Disease Control and Prevention, 2008).

This study details information by gender, race/ethnicity, quality of life, and by levels of awareness from a specific ethnic/geographic group (Texas Department of Health, 2002). Awareness information is important to consider not only for the total number of participants, but also for the number relative to the size of the population in question. Therefore, when possible, illustrations are reported in tables and figures to illustrate this point. The illustrations report findings from women who are affected, and/or who could become infected with HIV/AIDS in a particular population. Comparing these results showed the relative difference of the burden of disease across groups with different population sizes and therefore, shows how HIV/AIDS disproportionately affects the African American community and other groups (Suggs, 1997).

The data about HIV/AIDS awareness was recorded from the questionnaires. An interval of three weeks or longer passed for collecting data from each city, until the required data results were collected; consequently, more data could have been collected from a larger population, while collecting data from other races as well. Similarly, risk behaviors making up the mode of exposure among more recent information remain unknown pending further research of the awareness about HIV/AIDS (Jackson-Gray, 1999).

The researcher concludes that the data in this study are theoretical assumptions, supported by findings from the participants. The data has been adjusted for reporting, by recording the information to validate the data collected from each participant. The readers are urged to be cautious with the extent to which they generalize theories from these findings, as the content has been researched for informational purposes. This area of awareness could benefit from further research in identifying and understanding awareness factors associated with acquisition and transmission of HIV/AIDS in the fight against the disease (Levin, Bull, & Stewart, 2001).

REFERENCES

Adefuye, S., Abiona, T., Balogun, J., & Durrel, M. (2009). HIV sexual risk behaviors and perception of risk among college students: Implications for planning interventions. *BMC Public Health, 9*(281). doi: 10.1186/1471-2458-9-281

Ahmad, W. (2009, July 10). *Protect yourself against the dreaded HIV and AIDS.* Retrieved from http://ezinearticles.com/?Protect-Yourself-Against-the-Dreaded-HIV-and-AIDS&id=2591094/

AIDS.gov. (2010). *Interests.* Retrieved from http://www.aids.org/?s= interest

AIDS.gov. (2009). *Prevention Programs.* Retrieved from http://www. aids.gov/agencies/prevention/

AIDS Outreach Center of Greater Tarrant County. (2009). *2008-2009 program/agency accomplishments: About us.* Retrieved from http://www.aoc.org/about.asp/

American Social Health Association. (2009). *HIV and AIDS.* Retrieved from http://www.ashastd.org/learn/learn_hiv_aids.cfm/

Aramrattana, A., Bozzette, S.A., Celentano, D.D., Falco, M., Hammett, T. M., Kozlov, A.P., et al. (2006). Preventing HIV infection among injecting drug users in high risk countries: An assessment of the evidence (institute of medicine report). Washington, DC: The National Academies Press.

Arthur, G., Bhatt, S., & Gilks, C. (2000). The impact of HIV/AIDS on hospital services in developing countries—Will service breakdown ensue? *AIDS Analysis Africa 10*(6).

Avert. (2009). *Averting HIV and AIDS.* Retrieved from http://www. avert.org/aidsstigma.htm/

Baleta, A. (2004). Widespread horror over killing of AIDS activist in South Africa. *Lancet, 353* (9147), 130-131.

Basu, I., Jana, S., Rotheram-Borus, M.J., Swendeman, D., Lee, S.J., Newman, P. & Weiss, R. (2004). HIV prevention among sex workers in India. *JAIDS, 36*(3), 845-852.

Bell, G. (1998). *Fact sheet: 10 things to know about HIV/AIDS.* Retrieved from the The body—The complete HIV/AIDS resource website: http://www.thebody.com/content/art33163.html/

Benjamin R. (2007). A personal leadership journey. *ABNF Journal,* 102-103.

Berkowitz B. (2004). Rural public health services delivery, promising new directions. *American J Public Health, 94*(10), 1678-1681.

Bertozzi, S., Padian, N.S., Wegbreit, J., DeMaria, L.M., Feldman, B., Gayle, H., et al. (2006). HIV/AIDS prevention and treatment. In G. Alleyne, J.G. Breman, M. Claeson, D.B. Evans, D.T. Jamison, A.R. Measham, et al. (Eds.), *Disease control priorities in developing countries* (2nd ed.). Washington, DC: Oxford University Press, World Bank.

Biology News. (2006). New HIV statistics indicate increasing toll of AIDS on African American community. *Biology News Net.* Retrieved from http://www.biologynews.net/archives/2006/11/17/new_hiv_statistics_indicate_increasing_toll_of_aids_on_african_american_community.html/

Biscaro, M. (2004). Self efficacy, alcohol expectancy and problem solving appraisal as predictors of alcohol use in college students. *College Student Journal, 38*(4), 541-551.

Boykin, K. (2005). The 'down low' in life and legend. *Gay & Lesbian Review Worldwide, 12*(6), 34-36.

Brown, H., Jones, M., & Craytor, W. (2009). *Alaska HIV Prevention Plan.* State of Alaska Department of Health and Human Services. Retrieved from http://epi.alaska.gov/hivstd/hppg/

Burden, B.C., & Klofstad, C.A. (2005). Affect and Cognition in Party Identification. Experiment. *International Society of Political Psychology, 26*(6). Retrieved from www.as.miami.edu/personal/cklofstad/pid_polpsych.pdf.

Cantu, M. (2003). *Mastering Delphi 7.* Alameda, CA: SYBEX.

Casey M.M., Blewett L.A., & Call, K.T. (2004). Providing health care to Latino immigrants: Community-based efforts in the rural Midwest. *American Journal of Public Health, 94*(10), 1709-1711.

Castro, A., & Farmer, P. (2005). Understanding and addressing AIDS-related stigma: From anthropological theory to clinical practice in Haiti. *American Journal of Public Health, 95*(1), 53-59. doi: 10.2105/AJPH.2003.028563

CDC. (2003). Advancing HIV prevention: New strategies for a changing epidemic—United States. *MMWR, 53,* 329-332.

CDC. (2004). *HIV/AIDS Surveillance Report, 16.* Retrieved from http://www.cdc.gov/hiv/topics/surveillance/resources/reports/2004report/default.htm/

CDC. (2007). HIV/AIDS and African Americans. Retrieved from http://www.cdc.gov/hiv/topics/aa/index.htm/

CDC. (2009). *HIV/AIDS Prevention Research Synthesis Project.* AIDS Education Global Information System. Retrieved from http://www.aegis.com/ni/topics/prevent.asp/

CDC HIV/AIDS Factsheet. (2008). *HIV/AIDS among African Americans.* Retrieved from http://www.cdc.gov/hiv/ *CDC HIV/AIDS resources/*

Census. (2007, July). U.S. Census Bureau, updated July 8, 2008. Retrieved from http://factfinder.census.gov/

Census Bureau. (2004). *Statistical abstract of the United States, 2004-2005: The National Data Book* (124th ed.). Washington, DC: The Census Bureau.

Centers for Disease Control and Prevention. (2008). Cases of HIV infection and AIDS in the United States, by race/ethnicity, 1998-2002. HIV/AIDS Surveillance Supplemental Report;*10*(1):5. Retrieved from http: //www.cdc.gov/hiv/stats/hasrlink.htm.

Centers for Disease Control and Prevention. (2005). HIV/AIDS among African Americans [fact sheet]. Retrieved from http://www.cdc.gov/hiv/topics/aa/resources/factsheets/aa.htm/

Centers for Disease Control and Prevention. (2008). Trends in HIV/AIDS diagnoses. *Morbidity and Mortality Weekly Report, 57*(25). Retrieved from www.cdc.gov/mmwr/PDF/wk/mm5725.pdf/

Chafe R. (2004). *What approach should the providence take to primary healthcare reform?* Retrieved from http://www.nlma.nf.ca/nexus/issues/spring_2004/ ardcles/ardcle_5.html/

Cicero, L., & Pierro, A. (2007). Charismatic leadership and organizational outcomes: The mediating role of employees' work-group identification. *International Journal of Psychology, 42*(5), 297-306. doi: 10.1080/00207590701248495

Clissett, P. (2008). Evaluating qualitative research. *Journal of Orthopedic Nursing, 12,* 99-105.

Coleman, G., & O'Connor, R. (2007). Using grounded theory to understand software process improvement: A study of Irish software product companies. *Information and Software Technology, 49,* 654-667.

Collaborative Institutional Training Initiative. (2005). Online Human Subject Ethics Education Program. Retrieved from https://www.citiprogram.org/

Collins, C.E., Whiters, D.L., & Braithwaite, R. (2007). The saved SISTA project: A faith-based HIV prevention program for black women in addiction recovery. *American Journal of Health Studies, 22*(2), 76-82.

Copenhaver, M.M., & Fisher, J.D. (2006). Experts outline ways to decrease the decade-long yearly rate of 40,000 new HIV infections in the U.S. *AIDS and Behavior, 10,* 105-114.

Cravero, K. (2006). In our own hands: SWAA—Ghana champions the female condom. *Quality/Candid/Quality, 17* (1-2).

Crepaz, N., Lyles, C., Wolitski, R., Passin, W., Rama, S., Herbst, J., . . . & Stall, R. (2006). Do prevention interventions reduce HIV risk behaviors among people living with HIV? A meta-analytic review of controlled trials. *AIDS, 20,* 143-157.

Creswell, J.W. (2002). *Educational research: Planning, conducting, and evaluating quantitative and qualitative research.* Upper Saddle River, NJ: Merrill Prentice Hall.

Creswell, J.W. (1994). *Research design: Qualitative & quantitative approaches.* Thousand Oaks, CA: Sage Publications.

Culshaw, R.V. (2006, March 3). Why I quit HIV. Retrieved from the LewRockwell website: http://www.lewrockwell.com/orig7/culshaw1.html/

Department of Health and Human Services (DHHS). (2003). Advancing HIV prevention: New strategies for a changing epidemic—United States. *MMWR, 53,* 329-332.

Dowdy, D.W., Sweat, M.D., & Holtgrave, D.R. (2006). Country-wide distribution of the nitrile female condom (FC2) in Brazil and South Africa: A cost effective analysis. *AIDS 20*(16), 2091-2098.

Drain, M. (2004). Quality improvement in primary care and the importance of patient perceptions. *Journal of Ambulatory Care Management, 24*(2), 30-46.

Dunham, M. (2007, December 5). *The African American HIV/AIDS.* Retrieved from www.cdcnpin.org/

Durgo, J.A. (2002). *"HIV/AIDS" is spreading without sex due to lack of public awareness.* International AIDS Conference. Retrieved from http://www.aidssociety.com/internationalaids.html/

Eliot, J., & Czarnolewski, M.Y. (2007). Development of an everyday spatial behavioral questionnaire. *The Journal of General Psychology, 134*(3), 361-381.

Farmer P., & Kleinman, A. (1989). AIDS as human suffering. *Daedalus, 118*(2), 135-160.

Fauci, A.S. (2009, April 15). *HIV/AIDS HIV infection in women.* National Institute of Allergy and Infectious Disease. Retrieved from http://www3.niaid.nih.gov/topics/HIVAIDS/Understanding/Population+Specific+Information/womenHiv.htm/

Fauci, A.S., Braunwald, E., Kasper, D.L., Hauser, S.L., Longo, D.L., & Jameson, L.J. (2008). Human immunodeficiency virus disease: AIDS and related disorders. In *Harrison's Online, Harrison's Principles of Internal Medicine* (17th ed., chap. 182}. Retrieved from http://www.accessmedicine.com/

Federal Ministry on Health. (2004). *National policy on HIV/AIDS.* Retrieved from www.fmoh.gov.sd/English/Health-policy/doc/National Policy HIV.pdf/

Forman, J., Creswell, J.W., Damshroder, L., Kowalski, C.P., & Krein, S.L. (2008). Qualitative research methods: Key features and insights gained from use in infection prevention research. *American Journal of Infection Control, 36*(10), 764-771. Freed, B. (2006, November 22). World AIDS Day events set awareness, accountability are themes for 2007. *Dallas Voice.com, 5*(22). Retrieved from http://www.dallasvoice.com/artman/publish/article_4022.php/

Gao, F., Bailes, E., Robertson, D.L., & Chen, Y. (1999). Origin of HIV-1 in the chimpanzee Pan troglodytes. *Nature, 397*(6718), 436-444.

Gebo, K.A., Fleishman, J.A., & Moore, R.D. (2005). Hospitalizations for metabolic conditions, opportunistic infections and injection drug use among HIV patients: Trends between 1996 and 2000 in 12 states, *Journal of Acquired Immune Deficiency Syndromes, 40*, 609-616.

Gerald, G., & Wright, K. (2008, February). *Saving ourselves. The state of AIDS in black America 2008 . . . and what we're doing about it.* Retrieved from the Black AIDS Institute website: http://www. sfaf.org/files/site1/asset/blackaidsinst-savingourselves.pdf/

Glaser, B., & Strauss, A. (1967). *The discovery of grounded theory: Strategies for qualitative research.* Chicago, IL: Aldine.

Global Campaign for Microbicides. (2006). Microbicides: A promising HIV prevention option for African American women. *The Global Campaign for Microbicides, 3*(06), Retrieved from http://www.sistersong.net/publications_and_articles/AfrAm Women_Microbicides_April06.pdf/

Goffman E. (1961). *Asylums: Essays on the social situation of mental patients and other inmates.* Garden City, NY: Anchor Books.

Goffman E. (1963). *Stigma: Notes on the management of spoiled identity.* Garden City, NY: Anchor Books

Goldblum, P. B., & Erickson, S. (2000). An excerpt from working with aids bereavement: A comprehensive approach for mental health providers. *The Body—the Complete HIV/AIDS Resource.* Retrieved from http://www.thebody.com/content/living/art852. html/

Goldsmith, L. (2005). *University of North Carolina Chapel Hill.* Grants on Health Services Dissertation Research. Access in the U.S. and Canada: A Qualitative Inquiry. PAR00-076.

Greenhalgh, T., & Taylor, R. (2008). How to read a paper: Papers that go beyond numbers (qualitative research). What is qualitative research? *BMJ Medical Publication of the Year.* Retrieved from http://www.bmj.com/cgi/content/extract/315/7110/740?eaf=/

Grinstead, O., Comfort, M., McCartney, K., Kimberley, K., & Neiland, T. (2008). Bringing it home: Design and implementation of HIV/ STD intervention for women visiting incarcerated men. *Center for AIDS Prevention Studies. 20*(4), 285-300. Retrieved from http://www.ncbi.nlm.nih.gov/pubmed/18673062.

Gritzmacher, D., Cody, D., Minick, P., & Sowell, R. (2007). Ethical decision making with post-exposure prophylaxis (pep): HIV/

AIDS' double edged sword. *Journal of Health Administration Ethics, 1*(2), 73-82.

Hairston, E., & Smith, L. (1983). Black and deaf in America. *Prevention, 20*(4), 285-300. Retrieved from ProQuest Educational Journals.

Hanna, D. B. (2007). AIDS-defining opportunistic diseases in the HAART era in New York City. *AIDS Care, 19*(2), 264-272.

Harding, R., Molloy, T., Easterbrook, P., Frame, K., & Higginson, I.J. (2006). Is highly active antiretroviral therapy associated with symptom prevalence and burden? *International Journal of STD & AIDS, 17*(6) 400-405.

Harries, A.D., Maher, D., & Nunn, P. (1997). Practical and affordable measures for protection of health care workers from TB in low income countries. *WHO Bulletin, 75*, 477-489.

Haynes, M., Chng, C. L., & Vosvick, M. (2008). *Depression in college students: Perceived stress, loneliness, and self-esteem. Primary prevention: sexual behavior among college students.* University of North Texas. Retrieved from www.unt.edu/cph/current.shtml/

Health Central. (2009). Symptoms Reference. *Health Encyclopedia.* Retrieved from http://www.healthcentral.com/ency/408/sympidxa.html

Health Scout Network. (2009, April 1). *Diseases and Conditions,* The Health Central Network, Inc.—Health Encyclopedia. Retrieved from http://www.healthscout.com/ency/68/101/main.html/

Heffner, C.L. (2004). Research methods. Test validity and reliability. *All Psych Online 3*(4), 1-2.

Herek, G. (2001). Focus on HIV/AIDS and stigma. *NASTAD HIV Prevention Bulletin*, II./

Hertel, G., Konradt, U., & Orlikowski, B. (2004). Managing distance by interdependence: Goal setting, task interdependence, and team-based rewards in virtual teams. *European Journal of Work and Organizational Psychology, 13*, 1-28.

Higgins, J.A., & Hirsch, J. S. (2007). "The pleasure deficit: Revisiting the 'sexuality connection in reproductive health. *Perspectives on Sexual and Reproductive Health, 33*(3), 133-139.

Hill, J., & Vosvick, M. (2008). *An exploration of the variance in forgiveness in HIV+ adults through stigma and social support.* University of North Texas. Retrieved from www.unt.edu/cph/current.shtml/

HIV/AIDS Policy Factsheet. (2005). *The HIV/AIDS epidemic in the United States, November 2005.* Kaiser Family Foundation. Retrieved from http://www.kff.org/

Hofmann, S., Mantell, J.E., et al. (2004). The future of the female condom. *Perspectives on Sexual and Reproductive Health, 36*(3), 120-126.

Holy Bible: Kings James Version (KJV). (1978). New York, NY: American Bible Society.

Hoy-Ellis, C.P., & Fredriksen-Goldsen, K.I. (2007). Is AIDS chronic or terminal? The perceptions of persons living with AIDS and their informal support partners. *AIDS Care, 19*(7): 835-843.

Houghton, J.D., & Neck, C.P. (2002). The revised self-leadership questionnaire: Testing a hierarchical factor structure for self-leadership. *Journal of Managerial Psychology, 17,* 672-692.

Houghton Mifflin. (2000). *American heritage dictionary of the English language* (4th ed.). Boston, MA: Peter Langston. Retrieved from www.langston.com/English

Hovanesian J.A. (2008, May). State of the art: Treatment prospects for herpes simplex disease. *Ocular Surgery News. 26*(9), 48-50.

Huba, G. J., Kuo, C.T., Melchior, L.A., Elavia, C.A., & Tharasri, T.L. (1998). A world-wide-web site for disseminating information about evaluating innovative HIV/AIDS programs. *NLM Gateway—A service of the U.S. Institutes of Health, (12)* 996. Retrieved from http://gateway.nlm.nih.gov/MeetingAbstracts/ma?f=102231938.html/

Ignorance. (n.d.). *The American Heritage® Dictionary of the English Language* (4th ed.) Retrieved from Dictionary.com website: http://dictionary.reference.com/browse/Ignorance/

Implication. (n.d.). Dictionary.com Unabridged (v 1.1). Retrieved from Dictionary.com website: http://dictionary.reference.com/browse/Implication/

Interaction Institute for Social Change. (2009). *Facilitative Leadership.* Tapping the Power of Participation. Retrieved from http://www.interactioninstitute.org/services/training/facilitative_leadership

Jackson-Gray, J. (1999). *The difficulties of women living with HIV infection.* Retrieved from www.heartintl.net/HEART/HIV/Comp/ThedifficultiesofwomAIDS.htm/

Johnson, E.B. (2007). *HIV/AIDS epidemic in Dallas-Fort Worth area. Floor statement (Congresswoman, 30th Congressional District).* Retrieved from http://www.house.gov/list/speech/tx30_johnson/morenews/HIVAIDSEpidemicin DallasFortWorthArea.html/

Jones, I. (1997, December). Mixing qualitative and quantitative methods in sports fan research. *The Qualitative Report* [On-line serial], 3(4). Retrieved from http://www.nova.edu/ssss/QR/QR3-4/jones.html/

Kaiser Family Foundation. (1998). *The untold story: AIDS and black American: A briefing on the crisis of AIDS among African Americans.* Survey of African Americans on HIV/AIDS. Retrieved from http://www.kff.org/hivaids/1372-afr_amerre.cfm?RenderForPrint=1/

Kirby, D., Obasi, A., & Laris, B.A. (2006). The effectiveness of sex education and HIV education interventions in schools in developing countries. *World Health Organization Technical Report Series, 938,* 103-341.

Konradt, U., AndreBen, P., & Ellwart, T. (2008). Self-leadership in organizational teams: A multilevel analysis of moderators and mediators. *First article, European Journal of Work and Organizational Psychology.* doi: 10.1080/13594320701693225

Kornegay Jr., E.L. (2004). Queering black homophobia: Black theology as a sexual discourse of transformation. *Theology and Sexuality, 11*(1), 29-51.

Kwon, E. (2007, January 1). *Rick Warren: Church must S.T.O.P. HIV/AIDS.* Christian Today. Retrieved from http://www.christiantoday.com/article/rick.warren.church.must.stop.hivaids/8920. Htm/

Langston University International Scholarly and Scientific Organization. (2006). HIV/AIDS: The triadic triplets. *Journal of Scholarly and Scientific Perspectives, 2* (Spring). http://www.lunet.edu/JSSPpercent20combinedpercent20wpercent20revision.pdf/

Leu, D.J., Kinzer, C.K., Coiro, J.L., & Cammack, D.W. (2004). Toward a theory of new literacy emerging from the Internet and other information and communication technologies. In R.B. Rudell & N.J. Unrau, N.J (Eds.), *Theoretical models and processes of reading* (5th ed., pp. 1568-1611). Newark, DE: International Reading Association.

Levin, B.R., Bull, J. J., & Stewart, F.M. (2001). Epidemiology, evolution, and future of the HIV/AIDS pandemic. *Centers for Disease Control and Prevention, 7*(3), Retrieved from http://www.cdc.gov/ncidod/eid/vol7no3_supp/levin.htm/

Louis, K. (2003). School leaders facing real change. *Cambridge Journal of Education, 33*(3), 371-382.

LoveToKnow, Corp. (2008). *Seropositive.* Your Dictionary.com. Retrieved from http://www.yourdictionary.com/seropositive/

Loewenson, R. (2001, June). *HIV/AIDS implications for poverty reduction.* United Nations Development Programme. Retrieved from www.undp.org/hiv.index.html/

Luquis, R.R., Garcia, E., & Ashford, D. (2003). A qualitative assessment of college students' perceptions of health behaviors. *American Journal of Health Studies, 18* (2/3), 156-164.

MacLean, M.S., & Mohr, M.M. (1999). *Teacher-researchers at work.* Berkeley, CA: National Writing Project, pp. 56-66.

Malebranche, D. J., & Wheeler, D. (2005). Is HIV prevention targeting men "living on the down low" an effective strategy for African Americans? *Journal of Rural Health, 9*(29). Retrieved from http://www.albany.edu/sph/coned/t2b2hivprev05.htm/

Malviya, A., Hasan, H., & Hussain, A. (2009). Correlation of CD4+ T cell count with serum zinc, copper and selenium in HIV positive individuals. *Internet Journal of Epidemiology, 6*(2), 3.

Mantell, J.E., Stein, Z.A., & Susser, I. (2008). Women in the time of AIDS: Barriers, bargains and benefits. *AIDS Education and Prevention, 20*(2), 91-106. Retrieved from ProQuest Education Journals.

Manz, C.C., & Neck, C.P. (2004). *Mastering self-leadership: Empowering yourself for personal excellence* (3rd ed.). Upper Saddle River, NJ: Pearson Prentice Hall.

Martin, C.D. (2007). "All Reality is socially constructed." Social Science Research. Retrieved from http://www.seas.gwu.edu/~mfeldman/csci110/summer07/social-research.pdf

Mason, C. (2006). What makes a good leader? *Primary Health Care, 16*(10), 18-21.

McMillan, J.H. (1996). *Educational Research Fundamentals for the Consumer* (2nd ed.). New York, NY: HarperCollins College Publishers.

Medscape. (2007). General medicine, 9(1), 8. Retrieved from http:// www.medscape.com/

Merriam, S.B. (1988). *Case study research in education: A qualitative approach* (1st ed.). San Francisco, CA: Jossey-Bass.

Merriam, S.B. (1998). *Qualitative research and case study applications in education* (2nd ed.). San Francisco, CA: Jossey-Bass.

Minge, T. (2008). *People living with HIV/AIDS.* PLWHA. Retrieved from http://www.hivsa.org.au/

Ministry of Health. (2003). *National Strategy for HIV/AIDS prevention and control to the year 2010 with vision to the year 2020.* Retrieved from www.who.int/hiv/ ARV-guidelines.pdf.

Morgan, J., & Shoop, S.A. (2003). Celebrity speak out—TLC provides FYI on HIV. *DrDonnica.com, 06(03),* Retrieved from http://www. drdonnica.com/display.asp?article=6540/

Mulama, J. (2007). Africa: Commonwealth event debates why AIDS wears the 'face of a woman.' Inter Press service, Johannesburg South Africa.

National Institutes of Allergy and Infectious Diseases. (2002). *Classes of anti-AIDS drugs and therapeutics.* Retrieved from http://www. niaid.nih.gov/daids/dtpdb/clasdrug.htm/

National Institutes of Health. (2007). HIV infection in women. *HIV/ AIDS, 11*(2). Retrieved from http://www3.niaid.nih.gov/

National Prevention Information Network. (2008). *Minority HIV/ AIDS research initiative to build capacity in black and Hispanic communities and among black and Hispanic researchers to conduct HIV/AIDS epidemiologic and prevention research (U01).* Retrieved from http://www.cdcnpin.org/

National Science Foundation. (2006, October 23). *Government Performance and Results Act (GPRA) and Program Assessment Rating Tool (PART) performance measurement validation and verification.* Retrieved from www.nsf.gov/pubs/2007/nsf0701/ pdf/20.pdf/

Neck, C.P., & Houghton, J.D. (2006). Two decades of self-leadership theory and research: Past developments, present trends, and future possibilities. *Emerald Group Publishing Limited, 21*(4), 270-295. doi: 10.1108/02683940610663097

Neuman, W.L. (2003). *Social research methods* (5th ed.). Upper Saddle River, NJ: Prentice Hall.

Newman, K. (2002). *Studies of welfare populations: Data collection and research issues. The right (soft) stuff: Qualitative methods and the study of welfare reform.* Retrieved from http://aspe.hhs.gov/hsp/welf-res-data-issues02/11/11.htm/

Okechukwu, C. (2009, August). *Testimonial Archive.* The Safe Haven Project. Retrieved from www.charityadvantage.com/safehaven/Archives-ThinkingCap.asp/

Olivier, R. (2004). *Inspirational leadership: Henry V and the muse of fire.* London, UK: Spiro Press.

Operario, D., Smith, C.D., & Kegeles, S. (2008). Social and psychological context for HIV risk in non-gay identified African American men who have sex with men. *AIDS Education and Prevention, 20*(4), 347-359. Retrieved from ProQuest Education Journal.

Ory, M. (2001). *Planning grants for HIV/AIDS prevention and treatment intervention in middle-aged and older populations.* Healthy people 2010. Retrieved from http://www.health.gov/healthypeople/

Ostergard, R.L. (2009). *HIV/AIDS and the threat to national and international security.* New York, NY: Palgrave Macmillan Ltd. Retrieved from http://www.palgraveusa.com/catalog/product.aspx?isbn=1403933235/

Palmquist, M. (2009). *Reliability & validity. How to measure survey reliability and validity,* Thousand Oaks, CA: Sage.

Pankhurst, J.O. (2008, June). What worked? The evidence challenges in determining the causes of HIV prevalence decline. *AIDS Education and Prevention 20*(30), 275-283, Retrieved from ProQuest Education Journal.

Peters, R.C. (2008). From stigma to survival. *Drug Discovery & Development 11*(12), 4.

Phan, K.T. (2007, October 10). Black church leaders mobilize to combat HIV/AIDS. *The Christian Post* Retrieved from http://www.christianpost.com/article/20071010/black-church-leaders-mobilize-to-combat-hiv-aids/index.html/

Podosyan, G.A. (2007, December 18). *Human immunodeficiency virus.* American Medical Network. Retrieved from http://www.health.am/topics/more/human_immunodeficiency_virus/

Population Services International. (2009). *Youth AIDS* faith based alliances. Retrieved from http://www.psi.org/hiv/fbo2.html/

Power, B.M. (1996). *What to do with what you've written. Taking note: Improving your observational notetaking.* York, ME: Stenhouse Publishers.

Prochaska, J.O., Diclemente, C.C., & Norcross, J.C. (1992). In search of how people change: Applications to addictive behavior. *American Psychologist, 47,* 1102-1114.

Quinn, S.C. (1993). AIDS and the African American woman: The triple burden of race, class, and gender. *Health Education Quarterly, 20*(3), 305-320.

RedOrbit.com. (2008, August 27). *College students lack knowledge about HIV testing.* Council of Education for Public Health. Retrieved from http://www.redorbit.com/news/health/1535193/college_students_lack_knowledge_about_hiv_testing/index.html/

San Francisco AIDS Foundation. (2009, January 8). Why should you get tested for HIV? Retrieved from www.sfaf.org/aids101/hiv_testing.html/

Saunders, M, Lewis, P. & Thornhill, A. (2003) *Research Methods for Business Students* (3rd edition) Harlow: Prentice Hall.

Serafimovska, B., Maxwell, N.I., & Roberts, T. (2007). HIV/AIDS prevention services: An assessment of provider's needs. *Human Investment Research & Education (Hire) Center, B07* (0911). Retrieved from www.hire.csuhayward.edu/hire/discpap/abstracts/B07-09-11.pdf/

Sidoti, L. (2009, August 8). Obama: Health overhaul key to economic recovery. The Associated Press. Retrieved from http://news.yahoo.com/s/ap/20090808/ap_on_go_pr_wh/us_obama_health_care/

Simon, M. (2006). *Dissertation and scholarly research: Recipes for success.* Dubuque, IA: Kendall Hunt Pub. Co.

Singer, M. &. Baer, H. (2007). *Introducing Medical Anthropology.* New York, NY: Rowman & Littlefield Publishers, Inc., pp. 201-208.

SinoFresh HealthCare. (2009). *Privacy.* Retrieved from www.sinofresh.com/privacy.html/

Smith, J.A., & Daniel, R. (2006). Following the path of virus: The exploitation of host DNA repair mechanisms by retroviruses. *ACS Chemical Biology, 1*(4), 217-226.

Stampley, C.D., Mallory, C., & Gabrielson, M. (2005). HIV/AIDS among midlife African American women: An integrated review of literature. *Research in Nursing & Health, 28,* 295-305.

Stigma. (2009). *The American Heritage® dictionary of the English language* (4th ed.). Retrieved from http://dictionary.reference.com/browse/Stigma/

Stratford, D., Ellerbrock, T.V., & Chamblee, S. (2007). Social organization of sexual-economic networks and the persistence of HIV in a rural area in the U.S.A. *Culture, Health & Sexuality, 9*(2), 121-135.

Strauss, A., & Corbin, J. (1998). *Basics of qualitative research: Techniques and procedures for developing grounded theory* (2nd ed.). Newbury Park, CA: Sage.

Suggs, D. (1997, July). *True Colors.* POZ Health Life & HIV. Retrieved from www.poz.com/articles/242_1737.shtml/

Tarakeshwar, N., Kalichman, S.C., Simbayi, L.C., & Sikkema, K.J. (2008). *HIV prevention needs: Primary prevention and prevention for people living with HIV/AIDS.* In: D.D. Celentano & C. Beyrer (Eds), *Public health aspects of HIV/AIDS in low and middle income countries.* New York, NY: Springer, 19-40.

Tavakol, M., Torabi, S., & Zeinaloo, A. (2006). Grounded theory in medical education research. *Medical Education Online, 11*(30). Retrieved from http://www.med-ed-online.org/

Telles Dias, P.R., Souto, K., & Page-Schafer, K. (2006). Long term female condom use among vulnerable populations of Brazil. *AIDS and Behavior, 10,* 67-75.

Texas. (2007). *The Lone Star State.* Retrieved from http://www.lone-star.net/mall/texasinfo/texas.htm/

Texas Department of Health. (2002). *2002 epidemiological profile.* Retrieved from www.rwpc.org/Publications/2002 epi report. doc/

The Body: The Complete HIV/AIDS Resource. (2010). *Who Gets HIV/AIDS in the United*

States. Retrieved from http://www.thebody.com/index/whogets.html

Toro, A. (2006). Multisectorial responses to HIV/AIDS. *American Journal of Public Health, 96*(6), 995-1000.

Trochim, W. (2006). *Social Research Methods Knowledge Base*. Internal Validity. Retrieved from http://www.socialresearchmethods.net/kb/intval.php

Trochim, W.M., Cabrera, D.A., Milstein, B., Gallagher, R.S., & Leischow, S.J. (2006). Practical challenges of systems thinking and modeling in public health. *American Journal of Public Health, 96*, 538-546.

Tuan, N. (2006). Young African American women and HIV: Young African American women suffer a disproportionate impact of HIV and AIDS. *Journal of Advocates for Youth, 1*(1) 1-2.

Turner, S.M., DeMers, S.T., Fox, H.R., & Reed, G.M. (2001). APA's guidelines for test user qualifications: An executive summary. *American Psychologist, 56*, 1099-1113.

UNAIDS. (2007). *Confidentiality and security of HIV Information*. Retrieved from http://www.unaids.org/en/KnowledgeCentre/HIVData/Confidentiality/

UNAIDS. (2005). *Intensifying HIV prevention: UNAIDS policy position paper*. Retrieved from http://www.unaids.org/

UNAIDS. (1997). *Point of view women and AIDS*. Retrieved from data.unaids.org/Publications/IRC-pub02/JC750-Paediatric—PoV_en.pdf/

United Nations. (2001). *Joint communiqué from Secretary General and seven leading research-based pharmaceutical companies on access to HIV/AIDS care and treatment* (UN Press Release). Retrieved from http://www.un.org/

United Nations Economic Commission for Africa and UNAIDS. (2003, October 3). *Gender and HIV/AIDS: Leadership roles in social mobilization*. Retrieved from http://www.genderandaids.org/modules.php?name=News&file=print&sid=228/

USAID. (2009, July 2). *The U.S. government is the world leader in responding to the global pandemic of AIDS*. Retrieved from http://www.usaid.gov/our_work/global_health/aids/

U.S. Department of Health and Human Services. (2009). *Women & HIV/AIDS*. Retrieved from http://www.womenshealth.gov/hiv/

U.S. Department of Health and Human Services. (2006). *Comprehensive family assessment guidelines for child welfare*. Washington, DC: Administration for Children and Families Children's Bureau.

U.S. National Library of Medicine. (2009, June 8). *Fact sheet: AIDS information resources.* Retrieved from www.nlm.nih.gov/pubs/factsheets/aidsinfs.html/

Vu, M. (2007). *The Christian Post.* Obama Points to Rick Warren, T.D. Jakes as Models for Faith-Driven Action. Retrieved from http://www.christianpost.com

Warren, C.A.B., & Karner, T.X. (2005). *Discovering qualitative methods: Field research, interviews, and analysis.* Los Angeles, CA: Roxbury.

WHO. (2007). *WHO and UNAIDS announce recommendations from expert consultation on male circumcision for HIV prevention.* Retrieved from http://www.who.int/

Wilson, P. (2010, January 29). Black AIDS. In This Issue: Health Reform's Impact on People with HIV/AIDS. Retrieved from http://www.blackaids.org

Wingood, G. M., & DiClemente, R.J. (2006 August). Enhancing adoption of evidence-based HIV interventions: Promotion of a suite of HIV prevention interventions for African American women. *AIDS Education and Prevention 18* (4, Suppl A), 161-170.

Winter, G. (2000, March). A comparative discussion of the notion of 'validity' in qualitative and quantitative research. *The Qualitative Report,* 4(3/4). Retrieved from http://www.nova.edu/ssss/QR/QR4-3/winter.html/

World Bank, (1997). Confronting AIDS public priorities in a global epidemic. New York, NY: Oxford University Press.

World Health Organization. (2007). *AIDS epidemic update.* Retrieved from http://globalhealth.org/hiv_aids/

World Health Organization. (2005). *HIV/AIDS epidemiological surveillance.* Retrieved from www.who.int/hiv/pub/epidemiology/hivinafrica2005e_web.pdf/

Yammarino, F. J., Dionne, S.D., Chun, J.U., & Dansereau, F. (2005). Leadership and levels of analysis: A state-of-the-science review. *Leadership Quarterly, 16,* 879-919.

Yellin, T. (2006). Out of control. *Florida Public Health Review,* 2009; 6,14-18. Retrieved from http://health.usf.edu/publichealth/fphr/index.htm/

Yu, D., Souteyrand, Y., Banda, M.A., Kaufman, J., & Perriens, J.H. (2008). Investment in HIV/AIDS programs: Does it help strengthen health systems in developing countries? *Globalization and Health*, 4(8). doi: 10.1186/1744-8603-4-8

A P P E N D I X   A

DEMOGRAPHICS

First Name (Identifier Only):_____

Gender:_____Age (18-54)_____

Community (Dallas, Texas or Fort Worth, Texas):_____

Community College Student Fulltime or Part-time:_____

Race/Ethnicity:_____

Religion Preference or None:_____

Educational Level: Degree Program or

Continuing Education_____

Occupation:_____

Marital Status:_____

HIV Test History: Have Received or Never Received

HIV/AIDS Test:_____

Personal Relationship with HIV+/AIDS persons

(Family, etc.):_____

A P P E N D I X   B

INFORMED CONSENT

D. M. Dissertation Research Project
A Study of Lack of HIV/AIDS Awareness Among
African American Women

IRB approval # _____

Student Name: Betty Ragsdale   D. M. (Doctor of Management
                                       Candidate)
University of Phoenix 05/16/2009
Phoenix, AZ School of Advanced Studies

Description of Study:

The purpose of this qualitative grounded theory study will explore the lack of HIV/AIDS awareness in women in the Dallas and Fort Worth areas of Texas. Potential benefits from the study include a better understanding about the devastating disease of HIV/AIDS in the Dallas and Fort Worth areas of Texas. Information related to the University of Phoenix's questionnaire will be gathered by having the participants fill out an informed questionnaire or by interviewing the participant for approximately 15-30 minutes. The participants will be identified as Participant 1 and Participant 2 in order to protect confidentiality. The process will continue, until 30 participants have agreed to participate in this current study.

Cost and Payments to the Participant:

There is no cost and no payment for participation in this study.

Risk to the Participant:

There is no risk in participating in this study. This study is humbly submitted with respect, ethical principles, beneficence (no harm), and justice on a volunteer basis.

Confidentiality:

Information obtained in this study is strictly confidential. In addition, any information that can identify the participants will not be recorded, or used in any way to gain benefit for the research. The participants information will be labeled as Participant 1 and Participant 2, etc. The participants names will not be collected, and the (name space) on the questionnaire will be replaced with alpha/numeric numbers to protect confidentiality through the duration of the research, and after completion. In order to follow the University of Phoenix's informed consent procedures and protect the human subject, an alpha/numeric identifier will be assigned (e.g., 052209AB) to identify a participant, and the participants names will not be revealed in order to protect the participants contribution to the research.

Voluntary Consent by Participant:

Participation in this research study is voluntary, and consent is required before the research participant can participate in the research study. If, there is new information related to this study, the researcher will alert the participants immediately. The contact information should be placed public areas at local community colleges, and there will be a local telephone number listed for all participants to reach the researcher.

Participant's Right to Withdraw from the Study:

The participant may choose not to participate or to stop participation in the research program at any time without penalty. If the participant chooses not to participate, the information collected will be destroyed immediately, with the use of a paper shredder.

*   *   *

I have read the preceding consent form, or it has been read to me. I fully understand the contents of this document and voluntarily consent to participate. All questions concerning this research have been answered appropriately. I hereby agree to participate in this research study. Any questions regarding this study, please contact the doctoral researcher at a telephone number that will be provided. A copy of this form will be given to the participant. The return of this form with your alpha/number identifier will serve as your consent to participate in this study. The participant, not the researcher will select a random selection of alpha/numeric identifiers in order to minimize risks and gain trust from the participants.

Research Participant's Identifier: _____ Date: _____
Doctoral Candidate's Signature: _____ Date: _____

APPENDIX C

PERMISSION TO USE PREMISES

PERMISSION TO USE PREMISES
FOR THE UNIVERSITY OF PHOENIX, DOCTORAL
(STUDENT) RESEARCH

What is the purpose of this form? The community college and/or legal representatives are being asked to sign this form so that IRB/ARB may release me as a doctoral student to collect information on social and/or behavioral research. Participation in research is voluntary. If the Eastfield Community College and/or Tarrant County College choose to participate in the research and/or consent to permit the researcher to collect data from college students, a representative must sign this form, so that a certain population of students may be used in this research. The specific population and demographics of students are indicated on the potential questionnaire that will be used in this research.

    Participant Name: Eastfield Community College and/or Tarrant County College

IRB/ARB Approval Number:

Research Protocol: Open-Ended Questionnaires

Principal Investigator: Betty L. Ragsdale

Sponsor: University of Phoenix

What social/behavioral information does the researcher want to use? All social and/or behavioral information used in this study will be collected from college students; and the information will be used for community reporting purposes only.

Why does the researcher want social/behavioral information? The researcher wants to use this information as part of a research study entitled: A Study of Lack of HIV/AIDS Awareness Among African American Women.

Who will disclose, use, and/or receive this research information? The communities in Texas, especially the Dallas and Fort Worth areas, will disclose and use the research information. The recipients in African American communities, the Institutional Review Board (IRB) at the University of Phoenix, its representatives, surrounding communities, churches, and such agencies will receive this information.

How will this social/behavioral information be protected once it is given to the research sponsor? The information that is given to the study sponsor will remain private to the extent, and after extent of this study, as the study sponsor is required to follow human subjects federal privacy laws. Title 45 Code of Federal Regulations Part 46: Protection of Human Subjects.

How long will this informed consent: permission to use Dallas and Tarrant county premises last? The informed consent for the uses and disclosures described in this consent will not expire, as the information may be reported in the future, and will not warrant an expiration date. The collected data will be retained for; up to two years, and then, the information will be shredded to protect confidentiality.

The Informed Consent to use Premises for Research may be cancelled. You may cancel this informed consent to use premises at any time by notifying the study sponsor. If you choose to cancel this informed consent to use premises, the study sponsor will immediately stop all research questionnaires at your college. The researcher may continue to use the social/behavioral information that was provided before your college cancelled this informed consent to use premises.

Can the participants review the collected research information? The participants will have a right to request to see the outcomes/results of the collected research information. To ensure the scientific integrity of the research, the participants/community college representatives will not be able to review the research information until after the research study has been completed.

Check all that apply:

☐ I hereby authorize Betty L. Ragsdale; a doctoral student of University of Phoenix, to use the premises at (Eastfield Community College/Dallas, County) to conduct a study entitled A Study of the Lack of HIV/AIDS Awareness among African American Women: A Leadership Perspective.

☐ I hereby authorize Betty L. Ragsdale; a doctoral student of University of Phoenix, to use the premises at (Tarrant County College/Tarrant, County) to conduct a study entitled A Study of the Lack of HIV/AIDS Awareness among African American Women: A Leadership Perspective.

☐ I hereby authorize Betty L. Ragsdale; a doctoral student of University of Phoenix, to recruit subjects for participation in a conduct a study entitled A Study of the Lack of HIV/AIDS Awareness among African American Women: A Leadership Perspective.

☐ I hereby authorize Betty L. Ragsdale, a doctoral student of University of Phoenix, to use the name of the facility, organization, university, institution, or association identified above when publishing results from the study entitled A Study of the Lack of HIV/AIDS Awareness among African American Women: A Leadership Perspective.

Signature of University of Phoenix
Doctoral Student: _____ Date:_____

Signature of Community
College Representative: _____ Date:_____

Printed Name of College
Representative: _____ Date:_____

Position/Job Title of Authorized
Representative: _____ Date:_____

PERSONAL COMMUNICATION/ TELEPHONE INTERVIEW

Personal Communication/Telephone Interview
6/2/2009 9:35 p.m. Dr. Klinger/Dallas, Texas
214-660-7210

In this country, HIV/AIDS is a treatable Chronic Illness.

Betty Ragsdale's Question: Why do persons who have contracted the HIV/AIDS virus not tell their immediate family, but associates and friends ONLY?

Dr. Klinger's Response:
They are afraid
They will be disowned
Disappointment

Betty Ragsdale's Questions to the physician:
Is it common that those infected with the HIV/AIDS virus do not tell their parents?

Dr. Klinger's Response:
Yes. Prejudice against the fact . . . they would say, you must have done something wrong to get the HIV virus.

Dr. Klinger states: The virus affects the Endocrine System. The endocrine systems are fighting glands; they are composed of many glands such as the T-Cell, and Phagocytes, which are fighting within your body to fight off the virus. In addition, a

CBC—Complete Blood Count, does not show that a person has HIV/AIDS. In order for a physician to accurately determine and properly diagnose a patient, they must order a blood test by the name of CD-4 Test.

This test gives the total WBC (White Blood Count)

With the results, the physician is looking for the HIV antibody.

The physician will order an ELISA Test by way of:

Blood, Saliva, or Urine.

Further, the physician will order a blood test by the name of Western Blot, which confirms the diagnosis that also determines the stage of the disease.

Per Dr. Klinger, most females between the ages of 20-22 years are diagnosed when they are pregnant, because an AIDS test is required.

All it takes is sex (1) one time to get AIDS. Per Dr. Klinger, the HIV virus is in the population therefore, it is "out there" and you can get it.

Next, Dr. Klinger spoke about how many women who are married have contracted the HIV/AIDS virus. They have contracted the virus, because their spouses have cheated on them. Dr. Klinger's final statement was "There are a number of women who have the virus and it was contracted from their own husbands."

APPENDIX E

LEADERSHIP QUESTIONNAIRE

Leadership Questionnaire for the Days of Study   Date:_____

1. Behavior focused strategies:

    1. My goal for today is professionalism, research, writing, and staying focused.
    2. Have I accomplished it fully (scale of 1-5, maximum achievement marked as 5).
    3. What else could I have done better_____.

2. Natural rewarding patterns:

    1. Did I enjoy myself? If not, why?_____.
    2. What should I have done to enjoy my research?_____.

3. Constructive thought pattern:

    1. Did I visualize success?_____.
    2. Did I talk myself out of the difficulty faced today?_____.
    3. Did I correctly evaluate the ethical problems and act accordingly (scale of 5 and 5 for good performance)? _____.
    4. What else should I have done to improve my leadership behavior?_____.

4. Acceptance by research participants:

    1. Has the responses from the participants been good today?
        _____.
    2. Did they have any questions or concerns about the questionnaire?_____.
    3. If so, how did I respond to them?_____.
    4. My rate on a scale of 1-5, for my success with today's participants (% for maximum success)._____.

Satisfaction Rate on scale of 1 to 5 (5 for fully satisfied)—Summary of self-assessment.

SURVEY INSTRUMENT

QUESTIONNAIRE FOR PARTICIPANTS

The purpose of this survey presents an opportunity to solicit information about HIV/AIDS awareness among African American women.

Instructions:

- ~~Strike through~~ the most fitting response or level of awareness.
- Please answer questions from your perspective as an African American woman.
- Your individual information and responses will be kept confidential.

Thank you for participating in this study.

The sources for some of the questionnaire concepts are from E-Health Impact Study Questionnaire (2005).

1. ~~Strike through~~ the modes of transmission not possible for spreading HIV/AIDS by crossing out or striking through the alphabets at the beginning of the line.

a. Sharing needles to shoot drugs
b. Infected pregnant woman to unborn baby
c. Treated infected woman to her unborn child
d. Sexual intercourse with condom
e. Sexual intercourse without condom
f. Having sex with drug user who uses needles
g. Sharing tattoo needles
h. Becoming blood brothers/blood sisters
i. Sharing razor with someone who is HIV positive
j. Mother to baby via breast milk
k. Using public toilet seats
l. Being in same room with HIV person
m. Washing clothes with clothes of HIV positive
n. Passing HIV infection in the air like a cold
o. Kissing HIV infected person

2. Strike through the statements that you believe are wrong by crossing the alphabets at beginning of the line.

a. Safe to pick discarded needle or syringe
b. Being married prevents one from getting HIV and/or AIDS
c. Lower chances of infection by using latex condom
d. Lower chances of infection by taking birth control pills
e. Get HIV infection from donating blood.
f. Less chance of infection by using oil-based lubricants with latex condom
g. Lower chances of infection by having anal intercourse
h. Teenagers are more at risk than adult women.
i. You can get HIV infection from having blood test, so do not do a blood test.
j. Exchanging needles among family will not give you HIV infection.
k. Doctor always tests for HIV during blood test

3. Strike through the statements that you believe are wrong by crossing the alphabets at beginning of the line.

a. AIDS stands for acquired immune deficiency syndrome

    b. A healthy looking person can have AIDS.
    c. Infection with HIV can lead to AIDS
    d. HIV/AIDS attacks the immune system
    e. Vaccine can prevent from getting HIV infection
    f. There is a cure for the HIV infection
    g. Can have HIV for many years without knowing it
    h. All gay men have HIV/AIDS
    i. Person with HIV/AIDS live ten years or more
    j. Can get TB from HIV infected person with TB
    k. One who has HIV will get AIDS within two years
    l. One can get Gonorrhea and HIV at the same time
    m. HIV is easier to acquire than other STDs

4. Write an answer to the following questions:

    a. Number of concurrent sex partners?
    b. Ever been forced or frightened into sex?
    c. Have you always asked your partner to use a condom?
    d. Are you consistently protected with condoms, male or female? Yes or No.
    e. Type of sex in last 12 months. You can mark more than one if necessary.

        i) Unprotected vaginal sex
        ii). Unprotected oral sex
        iii) Unprotected anal sex

    f. Do you as a woman always negotiate your right to have safe sex?
    g. Does being married make your sex activity safe?
    h. Do you know how to assess that your partner has HIV/AIDS? If yes; how?
    i. Are you able to recognize symptoms of opportunistic infections?
    j. Have you discussed HIV/AIDS with your family?
    k. Does medical treatment cure AIDS?
    l. Does any good come out of taking treatment?
    m. Can you afford to take therapy if necessary?

n. Can an uninsured person take treatment?
o. Have you been covered by any preventive programs or helped by support groups?
p. If so, were you happy with what they offered?
q. If you had any complaints, what are they?
r. As being part of the African American community, what do you feel are the reasons for the large incidence of this dreaded disease in this community?
s. What could be done to reach maximum preventive help to you?
t. Have you used the diaphragm or female condom to protect yourself?
u. Have you had to look after an HIV infected person?
v. Is AIDS a chronic (having long duration) or terminal (causing the end of life:) disease?
w. How long does a person with new HIV infection progress to full-blown AIDS with treatment?
x. How will you save yourself from HIV/AIDS?
y. Who are the leaders in your community with knowledge about the cause of AIDS?
z. Have you been approached by these community leaders?

Thank you for completing this Questionnaire!